Unveil the Past, Heal the Future Through Hypnotherapy

Dolores Small Proiette, DCH, Ph.D.

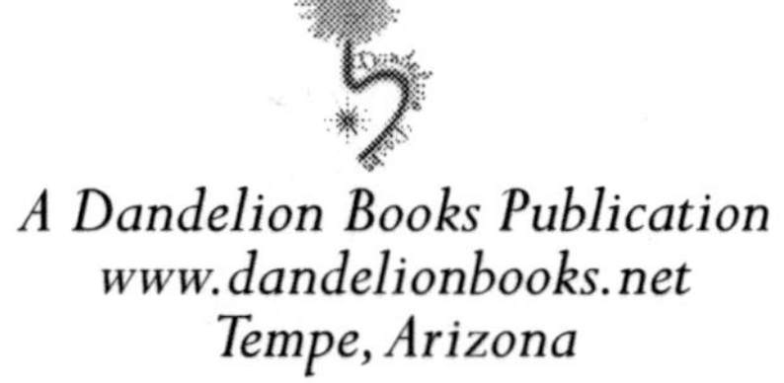

A Dandelion Books Publication
www.dandelionbooks.net
Tempe, Arizona

Unveil the Past, Heal the Future Through Hypnotherapy

A Dandelion Books Publication
Dandelion Books, LLC
Tempe, Arizona
www.dandelionbooks.net

Library of Congress Cataloging-in-Publication Data

Proiette, Dolores Small, DCH, Ph.D.

Unveil the Past Heal the Future Through Hypnotherapy

Library of Congress Catalog Card Number LC 2006936665

ISBN 978-1-893302-96-9, 1-893302-96-2

Cover and book design by Tjpublish, *www.tjpublish.com*

Disclaimer and Reader Agreement

Under no circumstances will the publisher, Dandelion Books, LLC, or author be liable to any person or business entity for any direct, indirect, special, incidental, consequential, or other damages based on any use of this book or any other source to which it refers, including, without limitation, any lost profits, business interruption, or loss of programs or information.

Though due diligence has been used in researching and authenticating the information contained in this book, Dandelion Books, LLC and the author make no representations as to accuracy, completeness, currentness, suitability, or validity of any opinions expressed in this book. Neither Dandelion Books, LLC nor the author shall be liable for any accuracy, errors, adequacy or timeliness in the content, or for any actions taken in reliance thereon.

Reader Agreement for Accessing This Book

By reading this book, you, the reader, consent to bear sole responsibility for your own decisions to use or read any of this book's material. Dandelion Books, LLC and the author shall not be liable for any damages or costs of any type arising out of any action taken by you or others based upon reliance on any materials in this book.

Printed in the United States of America

To my husband Vince, who has always been a positive and encouraging presence in my life, and to my daughters Kelly, Kari, and Kristi for their continual support.

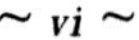

CONTENTS

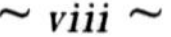

Foreword

I have read many books on hypnosis and hypnotherapy but none like the book you now hold in your hands. As a lay person and a trained hypnotist myself; and both a longtime practitioner and teacher of meditation—with years of working with the human heart and mind—I am greatly impressed with the invaluable information contained between these covers. *Unveil the Past, Heal the Future Through Hypnotherapy* is such compelling reading. Quite honestly, I found it hard to put down, and I believe this will be the case with most who have the privilege of reading it.

Dolores Proiette, DCH, Ph.D., through the use of carefully recorded and meticulously transcribed audio tapes, artfully and unwittingly draws the reader into the life of each of her patients. Through Dr. Proiette's superb and skillful hypnotic induction skills each person is lovingly led to search for and find the often obscure and sometimes extraordinary origins of their suffering.

Although the good doctor does not push the theory of reincarnation on anyone, she does refer to it in cases where the hypnotized patient encounters past life experiences or information. Rather than to speak in absolutes about such experiences, Dr. Proiette tells the reader that the mind of the patient may have created a metaphor or its own story to heal itself. Dr. Proiette has found, with many patients, that the emergence of such past life revelations is invaluable because such awareness, in her experience, often liberates a person from suffering in their present life.

Perhaps you will come to recognize some of your own story as the hidden inner realities of these precious patients' lives unfolds throughout the book. Afterwards you may even be eager to undergo—by way of a skillful and licensed hypnotherapist—some sessions to find the source of unmitigated suffering or some anomaly in your own life.

I was deeply honored to be asked by the author, a personal friend, colleague, and my own personal hypnotist, to write the foreword to a book that is so extraordinary and timely. It is must reading for everyone, including those who specialize in the field of psychology, or for any other health practitioner who wants to use or is using hypnotherapy as a modality for unlocking and healing the human heart, mind, and body.

A therapist in the field of hypnosis for over thirteen years, Dr. Proiette brings a wealth of experience and knowledge with her, though she writes in an uncomplicated and non-esoteric fashion. For those who have studied the work of the late Milton H. Erickson, M.D. par excellence, classical and world renowned psychiatrist, family counselor, and hypnotherapist, Dr. Proiette's approach and work seems very much like his. Not the least of which is her deep compassion and care that enable her to meet people (as Erickson did) where they are—without judgment—and take them where they need to be. She is, indeed, a very talented and loving person as a human being and in her chosen role of hypnotherapist to many.

The need for healing is universal and the means are multiple, but the use of hypnosis in the hands of a highly skilled hypnotherapist can easily and quickly surpass other approaches in getting down to the very root causes of much of human suffering. *Unveil the Past, Heal the Future Through Hypnotherapy* will help readers to more deeply appreciate hypnosis as it is applied for the alleviation of human suffering.

Philip K. Burley

Hypnotist, psychic intuitive, teacher of meditation, and author of *To Master Self Is To Master Life* and *A Legacy of Love, Volume I*

Introduction

"Be hypnotized? Are you kidding? No one's going to hypnotize me and make me act like a fool or say something I don't want to say," I thought. The word hypnosis brought up a fear of giving away my control, yet here I am almost two decades later with a doctorate in hypnotherapy asking others to accept something I once mistrusted. But I'm getting ahead of myself.

In my early forties, for many reasons, it was time I changed careers, and psychology always held my interest. But to do this I needed a college education, and up to this point my only college courses were non-credit courses that I took just for fun. I enrolled at the local community college taking courses during the day while my children were in school. I soon added one night course a week at a local university that was geared toward adult students. During an oral report in my psychology class, as I touched on an event that happened to me in the fifth grade, I began choking and stammering trying to hold back the tears. I couldn't believe it, where was this coming from? The teacher was quite forgiving deciding she would read the rest of my report quietly. After much questioning on her part after class, she said that my "breakdown" was deeper than was seen on the surface. Being a psychologist, she suggested I come to her office the next day.

After further discussion in her office, she decided to hypnotize me. Her gentleness alleviated any fears I had about hypnosis, so we began. I remember thinking, "I'm not hypnotized. Why are you asking me questions? Can't you see I'm not hypnotized?" Yet with each question she asked, I responded, not understanding from where the information was coming.

I saw myself standing in a crib wearing a one-piece white outfit. I was eight months old, happy and bouncing while I held onto the crib railing. There was a figure dressed in black next to my crib with its back to me. The figure's hair was short, light in color, and smooth. As I was asked to have the person turn around, I kept saying, "No, I can't turn it around." Finally, after much prodding, I turned the figure around only to see a disfigured witch's face! I was stunned, yet realized it was my mother who actually was a beautiful looking woman. As my father appeared in the doorway, a terrible fear came over me. I saw my mother put me in a closet and close the door. The scene that unfolded was my father telling my mother that she would never put me in the closet again, and then a terrible fight ensued.

I felt drained after the session. What happened can't be, I thought. I had to call my mother.

As soon as I got home, I called her. "Mom, did you put me in a closet when I was a baby?" I asked.

"What?" she replied.

I said, "I was just hypnotized and saw you putting me into a closet and closing the door. Did you do that when I was a baby?"

As she started giggling nervously, my mother said, "But you were so ugly, I didn't want anyone to see you. When people came to visit, if I put you in the closet maybe they wouldn't remember you were there and wouldn't ask for you, but I didn't close the door; I just put you behind it. I didn't do it for long because you got curly hair and started walking at such an early age and then you were so cute."

This made me a believer in hypnosis. I had no conscious awareness of what had happened as an infant, yet my mother was verifying it. I saw her with a witch's face because of the fear of the dark and closed spaces she instilled in me at such an early age. To take this a step further and understand where my mother was coming from would give understanding as to why I held no ill feelings towards her. She was the fourth of nine children, with the responsibility of caring for her younger siblings so both parents could work. As a result, even though she was young, she was tired and didn't want children of her own, but instead wanted a career as a model. She was a beautiful, tall woman with long, blonde hair, which she wore up in a chignon. My mom lived with her parents and cared for her younger siblings until she married at the age of twenty-six. Soon after, she became pregnant with me squelching her chances for becoming a model.

I went back to the psychologist for two more sessions, each one uncovering events I had "stuffed" deep within my subconscious unaware they were holding me back. After the third session, I noticed changes in myself. I no longer cowered when getting into a lively discussion with someone else. I stood up for myself and began liking myself. I was finally taking back my power. Fears I had developed over the years were gone. Now, I wanted to find out more about hypnosis!

I asked the teacher if she would instruct a class in hypnosis; it turned out to be a class in self-hypnosis, which I eagerly took. After that, I flew from Phoenix to Los Angeles on weekends taking classes at the American Institute of Hypnotherapy and becoming certified in hypnosis. I was on a roll and metaphorically speaking, "My door had been opened."

Within four-and-one-half years I had attended college and graduated with a doctorate, started my own business, and went through a divorce after twenty years of marriage while raising two daughters. Whew!

Hard work, yes, but I attribute much of my success to hypnosis, freeing me to move forward and be myself.

Hypnosis is useful and important in that the subject is enabled to connect directly with the subconscious where all past events that caused trauma are stored. In the process of remembering a traumatic event, energies tied to the memory can be released reducing therapy to months, weeks or days rather than years without the use of drugs that may have harmful side effects. The state of unrest or disease (a feeling of dis-ease within the body) connected with the memory is removed. This helps heal the body, mind, and soul, causing a transformation within the person. Such was the case of Evelyn in Chapter 3, who had been plagued with chronic pain in her left hip for several years. Since the hypnosis session three years ago, she has not needed chiropractic adjustment.

I do not impose my beliefs upon my clients. If they accept the premise of past lives, that's fine. If not, I suggest they imagine the subconscious creating a story in order to bring to the surface the cause of their emotional or physical problem. Metaphors are useful in hypnosis and can bring the same results as clients believing their "story" is a past life. However the information is brought forth, it's possible that the problem or pain can be removed or reframed.

In some cases by accessing a past lifetime as with Sally in Chapter 1, the client becomes aware of patterns carried into the current lifetime. In Sally's case, this allowed her to understand the issues she was facing, enabling her to be more compassionate with others around her. Sally's new insight gave her the tools to change the old patterns of her life.

Dolores Cannon, author and regressionist said:

> Everyone is constantly changing. Not to change would mean you have stopped growing. At that point you become stagnant and start to die. We change so much that many times we may feel as though we have lived many different lives in this one. We go to school, marry, have children, sometimes marry again. We may change occupations, sometimes going in an entirely different direction. We may travel or live in a foreign country for a while. We may experience trauma and sorrow with the death or unhappiness of loved ones. We hopefully learn to love and attain our goals in life. Each of these are stages in our lives and they are totally different from the other. We make mistakes and hopefully learn from them.

~ ~ ~

Many people have a fear of dying. Through the vehicle of hypnosis, we are able to access wisdom within. From that vantage point, we might be able to feel the unconditional love God has for his children. This could remove a fear of dying, allowing the subject to see death as transformative growth.

The hypnosis sessions that follow are those of a varied selection of clients transcribed from tapes made during the session. The names, locations, and other forms of identification have been changed to protect the clients, and on occasion several questions are combined into one to shorten the text.

Our deepest fear is not that we are inadequate.
Our deepest fear is that we are powerful beyond measure.
It is our light, not out darkness that most frightens us...
And as we let our own light shine,
We unconsciously give other people
Permission to do the same.
As we are liberated from our own fear,
Our presence automatically liberates others.

— Marianne Williamson

CHAPTER 1

HAVE WE MET BEFORE?

"Love is the most powerful force in the universe. Not time, birth, death, or rebirth can finally separate those who have formed a deep mental, spiritual, or physical bond. The soul's affinity has been established, and those who know or have known love will always be 'one,'" says Dick Sutphen, quoted as America's foremost psychic researcher, as he begins his book, *You Were Born Again to be Together*. He continues:

> Physical separation and parting for more than a short period of time, as we know it, is absolutely impossible. Mental separation is unknown on a subconscious level. Communication will always continue, although it may not be consciously perceived. Lovers from the past will reincarnate within the same time frame again and again. Although they will not remember events of their past lives when they meet in their next life, they will be strongly attracted to each other, and love will be renewed. People with whom you have a deep bond in this life have been close to you in a previous lifetime.

My mother sent me a copy of his book when it first came out in 1976. For whatever reason, I was unable to get past the first few pages, so I put the book on my shelf where it stayed for several years. I moved to Phoenix, Arizona, and while unpacking came across the book again. As the pages unfolded, I began reading and couldn't put it down until I had read the last page! There I was in the middle of all these boxes yet to be unpacked, and I stopped to read a book from cover to cover. Why? I don't know. Maybe I wasn't ready to acknowledge the information before, yet couldn't get enough of his books after that. I went to libraries and bookstores, reading every book he had written. Was this my subconscious introduction into the field of hypnosis?

The following hypnosis sessions indicate that love and friendship carry through lifetimes.

Joanne

This session occurred in 1998. Joanne was dating a friend of mine and when she heard I was a hypnotherapist, she called for a past-life regression session. She wanted to find out more about her connection with Donald, the man she had been seeing. As fate would have it, I believe the past-life regression was actually to re-connect Joanne and me – and more!

After she was put into a hypnotic state, I regressed Joanne back to a time when she and Donald were together:

D: Tell me where you are, in detail.

J: This looks like a crystal palace; everything is crystal. It's something silver on my feet; it's like silver boots and a long, silver, shiny, cheery-looking dress, with long sleeves. It looks almost futuristic, but it's not. Everything is really bright and crystal looking. Everywhere I look there are bright, silver, crystal lights. I can't really see my face; I just know I'm here.

D: What color is your hair?

J: Honey-colored. It's straight, kind-of shoulder length.

D: Are you male or female?

J: Female, and I have some kind of a silver band around my head with some sort of jewels on it. It's blue, sapphire-blue crystals. This place looks really strange. It's technical looking. Here, I'm going up these stairs. It just goes up and up and up and up. Amazing.

D: Continue following it up.

J: There's this room at the very top. It's very illuminated. There's a lot of people and they're all dressed similarly. I think it's a temple.

D: What's it called?

J: The first thing that came into my mind was Athena, but A-then-a-ah, something like that. Atlantia, Atlantia, that's what it is.

D: Where is it located?

J: I think I'm on Atlantis. Oh, God. On the top of the temple is like a glass ceiling, and there's all these stars. It's an observatory or something, where you can look at the stars. And they have a telescope. I don't know how they can have a telescope.

D: Just allow it to come out; you can analyze it later.

J: I'm looking through the telescope and we're charting, we're doing astrological things, like charts. I've got this big graph and I'm drawing the constellations. I'm charting something. I feel like the thing on my head, I can actually hear stuff through it. (Giggles.) You're right there. You're there. You just turned around and I saw you. You work in there, too. Oh, I love this place; it's really beautiful. It's bright and exciting and everybody is involved in the same kind of work. You've got a yellow diamond-shaped thing on your head. I recognized your eyes. You're real tiny, really tiny, and petite, with big brown eyes. There are a whole lot of people in here.

D: What is your name?

J: Or-i-on. You're coming over to me and we're taking this chart around to show to people there. This really feels happy in here. From this temple, you can see for hundreds of miles all around. It almost feels like it's spacey, I mean like the future. There's Donald, I found him. It's hard not to recognize that smile. He's got this kind of white robe-looking thing on. Actually, you do, too. You've got one that looks almost Grecianish.

D: What are our positions there?

J: We're all just technical people, and we each have a different – I don't know who the boss is.

D: Just follow it in time, to the next significant event.

J: It's like there's an earthquake, and everything is crumbling all over the place.

D: What year is it?

J: 15,000, I don't know, it's amazing. Oh, God, I have a stomach ache. This is really upsetting. Everything is falling apart. We're all running and we're holding hands. All the beautiful stuff is falling.

D: If you need to view it as a movie and separate yourself, then do so. But if you wish to be part of it and experience the emotions, that is your choice.

J: (Calms down.) We're running down this thing, and everything is crumbling everywhere. We're trying to get to the ship. There's the ship, at the bottom of this island. (Long pause.) Okay. We're on the ship. We're going through the fog.

D: Who's we?

J: Well, there's you and me and Donald, and some other people. I don't know who the other people are; they were on the island. There's a name, somebody named Patty, I don't know who she is. She's blonde. She keeps saying Patty to me, I don't know.

D: Go to the lady named Patty. In that time, was that her name? What is her name there in that lifetime?

J: Delphia.

D: Thank you. Continue.

J: We traveled a long time.

D: Where are we headed?

J: We're at an island; it's very misty. We're getting ready to disembark. There's about ten or fifteen people and it's very cold. There's a forest here. We're going to establish ourselves.

D: What is the name of the place?

J: Ire. Ire? Eir, Eire, something like that. It's just so green and some of us are starting to build some stone huts, which is a far cry from where we were.

D: When you boarded the ship, did you look back at Atlantis? What did you see?

J: It was all crumbling; it was all falling in.

D: Falling where?

J: Into the ocean. We were lucky we got away.

D: Did it disappear completely, or was there some left?

J: No, it's gone. Everything is gone.

D: Was that the last earthquake on Atlantis?

J: Yes, because it's gone. There's nothing there. This is very primitive compared to – it's like starting all over, and it's very cold here. We're just establishing a little community. And you're with a man, there's a man with you. I guess he's your – you sure look like you're together. His name is Phalo. You guys are so cute, you're so tiny and he's tall; he's really tall and long-limbed and blonde. He has kind of a Grecian-looking face. He's very protective of you, but he's a gentleman. He said Gerald, Jerry is his name.

D: What is Donald called?

J: Claudet, which is a very weird name.

D: What is your relationship with him?

J: I think we were engaged. We're engaged, betrothed as they called it then, betrothed. So we're building our – you've gone away, further away. You guys want to build your own place further away. It looks like a Loch. It looks like green mountains right by this water. There's a forest; it's really beautiful, but kind of cold, looks misty. The other people there, about fifteen people, they're all moving away, establishing their own place. The name came up here, Ire.

D: Ireland?

J: It could be Ireland, yes. It looks – I don't know what Ireland looks like, but this, it's really pretty. But there's nothing here, no people, just us.

D: Move forward to the next significant event.

J: We're really old. I don't like his name in this life; I'm going to call him something else.

D: What do you call him?

J: Clive. (Giggles.) Clive. He's got this long beard, long hair. His hair is way long and he looks really old. We don't have any kids. I can see houses down, miles away. We live up on a hill. And, you, you're married. You guys live down, closer to the water. You're getting old too, been here a long time.

D: As you are scanning that lifetime, what is the reason and purpose of that lifetime?

J: Oh, my goodness! We're doing some kind of ritualistic stuff, like a – some kind of a worship. Everybody is wearing long white robes. I don't know what's going on, but it seems like – to carry some spiritual ideas with us. That's what I'm getting from it.

D: Go into that in more detail, describe what that is all about.

J: It's trying to work with the mind, to encourage the mind in search of pursuits. We're all standing around in white robes trying to remember the things that we knew or brought with us, the astrological things and the higher spiritual things, that's what I'm getting. Your friend, is it your friend? She keeps saying she's your friend.

D: You mean Patty?

J: Yeah. (Sighs.)

D: Yes, she's my friend.

J: She is in the middle of all of this. She is the one who is instructing us, I guess that's what she's doing, or leading us somehow. She's quite pretty; she's not married. She's like a priest or something. She's teaching us, no, we already know this. She's not teaching us, she's instilling it. She wants to make sure it's not forgotten. That's what she's doing. Wait. We do this as a remembrance, to carry the things on that we knew, that's what she said, like a ritual. For some reason none of us have any kids. You don't and I don't. At this rate, this will die out.

D: Is there any information that you need to pass on to us at this time that we need to remember about the ritual?

J: Yes. We need to live in our hearts and our minds and learn to use our minds to touch others, to talk to them, to reach them, so that we can understand each other's thoughts, instead of misunderstandings. It's not very clear.

D: Take your time.

J: (Pause.) To learn to speak on alpha waves with each other, alpha waves.

D: How did we communicate during that time?

J: We're trying to practice this; we're doing this. Evidently we knew this before and it was accepted. Oh, that's what those things on our heads were for. It was an accepted way of being and because we've been disconnected from our culture, we've, like stepped backward. We're taking steps backward instead of forward, and we need to remember or to continue to practice this, and because we're so – before when we were on Atlantis we all lived together in one place in the temple, and we all talked to each other without talking. Then we lost that and we separated ourselves into little communities and we lost it. We need to remember this so we don't lose what we once had. That's why we meet ritualistically like this, to try to continue on with it.

D: Are there any suggestions for us to continue it in this lifetime, any specific instructions?

J: Develop our physic ability and rather than living in the physical, live in the spiritual. Practice it. Practice focusing on it in your mind and try to speak to people with your mind. I just feel like crying. That was a beautiful place, and it just disappeared. It's gorgeous.

D: Is there any other information you need to bring forth about that for yourself?

J: I'm definitely in the right place in this lifetime. I'm doing the work I should be doing, and I'm with the people I should be with. I just feel so sad about that beautiful place.

End of session.

After the session, Joanne became excited and said, "I'm going to go home and draw a picture; you just won't believe how beautiful it is. And your friend, Patty, she just kept jumping up and down from behind some people, saying, "It's me! Tell her it's me! She wouldn't shut up until I said her name."

Friendships travel through time and space lasting lifetime after lifetime. Patty and I had been close friends for more than six years when Joanne was hypnotized. What surprised me is that while Joanne was hypnotized, Patty's energy was so strong as to come through Joanne's session by saying, "She's a friend of mine," giving her current lifetime name, even though Joanne and Patty had not yet met in this lifetime. Several months later, I introduced Joanne to Patty. The three of us have been close friends ever since.

Equally startling, Gerald or Jerry is the name of my former husband of twenty years in this lifetime, of which Joanne had no knowledge.

ELLEN

Ellen, a lovely 17-year old, slowly followed her mother, Judy, into my office. It was a love-anger relationship between Judy and Ellen, which had become progressively worse over the past year. One day Ellen worshiped her mother, the next day she was belligerent and argumentative. Judy had a degenerative disease that would act up at times causing much pain. When this occurred Ellen would begin yelling and stomping out of the room. We later became aware this negative reaction was caused by a subconscious fear that Ellen's mother was going to die and leave her alone again.

After lengthy discussions, Ellen was eager at the thought of being hypnotized, something she could tell her friends about in school. When regressing Ellen back to the cause of the problems she and her mother were having related to Judy's illness, Ellen's subconscious went back into a lifetime where she was now an elderly man named Jim. He was on a cruise ship sitting on a lounge chair with a blanket wrapped around him. Nothing made him happy. He complained about the service being too slow, the children playing on board were noisy, it was too cold and damp, and so on. Jim was grouchy and unpleasant, stating he was waiting for his turn to die.

I moved him to an earlier time within that life. He was now eighteen years old, engaged to Beth, his fiancée. She was a beautiful young woman with golden blonde hair cascading from beneath her bonnet. She wore a long, full dress, her beautiful blue eyes gazing into his. Jim was standing next to her in a dark brown suit with tails. It was the 1800s and he was "on top of the world," so much in love with Beth. They were to be married in two weeks.

The following week Beth became sick and suddenly died from complications of her illness. Jim, irate at the fact that Beth left him, vowed he would never love again. He died at an old age, very lonely and bitter.

As it unfolded, Ellen was Jim; Judy was Beth. Still under hypnosis and looking at the situation from a higher conscious perspective, Jim was able to realize that Beth did not intentionally leave him; death was unwanted and unexpected by Beth. He was then able to forgive his fiancée.

The understanding of that lifetime allowed Ellen to dissolve the love/anger feelings for her mother and the subconscious fears of losing her beloved once again, which were growing stronger as she came closer to the age of eighteen.

I have had other clients with emotional trauma from the past that developed a phobia or fear as they neared the age of the original traumatic occurrence. Once the cause of the trauma is unveiled, the phobia or fear disappears.

TONYA

Love travels through time and space. A deep love relationship in one lifetime will carry into future lifetimes going to the core of one's soul. But what about timing, how does that factor into this lifetime?

"Why am I always doing this to myself," asked Tonya. As she sat in my office, I wondered about the outgoing personality I had recently talked to on the telephone. She was a young woman in her late twenties and strikingly beautiful. As she began talking, I felt that she was a woman who was concealing a deep pain and that she was alone in the world. She had recently gone through a divorce and was becoming involved with a man she had known when she was a teenager. Johnny was married with a small child, yet Tonya "could not stay away from him," she said. "I know it's not right and I've tried to stop seeing him, but that doesn't last long. I see him whenever I can, even if it's only a couple of hours at a time. Why am I hurting myself this way?" Tonya wanted to find out why this obsession with Johnny was emotionally harming her, Johnny, his family, and those around her.

As she was regressed to another lifetime, she began:

T: It's a beach – rocky beach, with really big waves. I'm standing there.

D: Look down at your feet. What do you see?

T: Sand.

D: Look up. What are you wearing?

T: White.

D: How do you feel as you stand there?

T: Sad.

D: What is causing you to feel sad?

T: The waves. (Sniffs.) I don't know why the waves make me sad, but they're big.

D: Allow yourself to walk forward along the beach. Tell me what you see. What's going on?

T: There's nobody there. It's dusk.

D: Why have you decided to come to the beach?

T: I live somewhere near there.

D: Allow yourself to go back to your house. Walk along the beach until you come to your house. Tell me what's going on.

T: It has to be a long time ago, because it's an older cabin. It looks like something you'd see in the movies. It's just one room.

D: What year is it?

T: Sometime in the 20's or 30's.

D: What are the feelings that come up as you walk around your cabin?

T: Somebody else built it for me.

D: How old are you?

T: Probably this age. I feel as though I look the same, I feel the same. Probably thirty.

D: What is your name?

T: (Giggles.) I want to say Esmerelda, but that's – (Giggles again.)

D: Just allow it to come forward. You can analyze it later. Allow yourself to move forward to a significant event; tell me what's going on.

T: (Begins sniffing.) I'm sitting on my bed, waiting and then a group of people, my friends, come to the door. They're all hugging me and crying and sitting on my bed with me. I'm just shocked.

D: What has caused you to be shocked?

T: They say my girlfriends have husbands that work with my husband. I think something bad happened.

D: Allow it to come forward. What happened to your husband?

T: They work on a boat, and only a few of them made it back. I think they're fishermen, but they've come to tell me that he didn't make it back. I don't believe them. I'm not crying. I want to cry, but I'm not crying.

D: Allow yourself to go back within that lifetime to a happy time. Tell me what's going on.

T: It's just the two of us. He's building me a house! I'm helping him. (Deep sigh.)

D: How do you feel when you're together?

T: Happy!

D: Walk up to him, feel his energy, look into his eyes. Do you recognize him as anyone in your current lifetime?

T: (Begins crying.) It looks so much like Johnny. He's just a little bigger, just a little bigger, like he's been working his whole life – a little rougher, and his skin is tanned, kind of leathery, but he has the same eyes.

D: Allow the scene to unfold.

T: He stops working; he's hugging me. I feel much smaller when he hugs me. He's – like the biggest man I've ever met, but he's not, and we're happy. I don't miss anything.

D: How old are you at that time?

T: Pretty close to, maybe a year younger, like we're just beginning our life together. I feel like we ran away from something.

D: Allow yourself to go back in time, just prior to having some problems in that lifetime. Allow it to unfold.

T: I feel like I had another, I had a family. He was – we lived in the city, we didn't live by the water. We always – we always saw each other, but I had a family.

D: What do you mean by you had a family?

T: I think I was married before, taking care of somebody. I had responsibilities, and I couldn't leave. We didn't even talk. We just smiled at each other all the time.

D: Continue going back in time within that lifetime to a significant event. Tell me what's going on.

T: My mother chose who I was going to marry. We all lived in the same house together.

D: Go up to your mother. Do you recognize her as someone in your current lifetime?

T: Yeah! My mother!

D: Now, go up to the man she chose that you were going to marry. Do you recognize him as someone in your current lifetime?

T: No.

D: Allow it to unfold. How old are you?

T: Maybe nineteen. This sounds weird, but I think my mom was with him, I don't know why.

D: Allow it to unfold; you can analyze it later as you go down, down, down.

T: (Long pause, coughs.) I think they were trying to kill me – my mother and my husband! (Begins coughing continuously.)

D: You can view it as a movie or go through the event again, it is your choice. Allow the scene to unfold and tell me what's going on.

T: (Calms down.) Yeah, they had started a relationship, and I heard them talking. Yeah, they were going to kill me, so I left. I didn't bring anything, I just ran. I went to find Johnny, who I hadn't even talked to, but I went and found him. He was working; it was nighttime. I found him and just grabbed him and we left that night – to the place we had been before, because it was what he did for a living. He worked on a boat. I don't know what he did, if he was a fisherman, but it was really hard work. He was always – just worn.

D: How old is he?

T: Maybe just a little older than I am.

D: Allow the lifetime to continue to unfold and tell me what's going on.

T: We stayed in a little room that we rented while we built our cabin. We were happy, so so so so so happy!

D: Was there anyone else in his life?

T: No, I feel like he was just waiting for me. Like just seeing me, just passing him on the street was enough. Like one day, maybe he knew that the situation I was in wasn't right.

D: What is the town called that you went to?

T: It's like – I want to say Bayport. I don't even know what that means. I feel like it's in the east somewhere, but it's small. Everybody there is really friendly. There aren't many children there, just a lot of men and women, and most of the men work on boats.

D: Go back to the time when your friends came over. Feel the essence of your friends; do you recognize any of them in your current lifetime? Take your time.

T: One looks like my Aunt Darla, and one looks like my dead friend, Corina. The others I don't recognize. There were only four or five.

D: Allow the years to unfold. Tell me what is going on.

T: I don't see myself. I stopped. I don't even talk to my friends; I don't even buy groceries. I don't know how I'm living; I'm just sleeping. I don't think it's been very long since he didn't come back, but everybody was talking like he wasn't going to come back. I just want to believe he's fine, but then I stand there and watch the waves hit the rocks and I think about his head.

D: Why do you think about his head?

T: I think that it's been smashed. There's no way. I don't have any hope.

D: Go to the time just before your death scene. How old are you?

T: I'm thirty.

D: Tell me what happens.

T: I jump off a really, really tall rock. But I don't feel bad about it because I don't have anything. I don't want anything. I was done. I was hoping somehow that our bodies would wash up together.

D: Scan your body. Where are you holding onto your pain of his leaving, his dying?

T: My chest.

(The pain in her chest was removed; she chose to fill the area with will and strength.) Whenever a negative energy is removed from the physical body, the area needs to immediately be filled with a positive energy; otherwise the person may later fill the area unintentionally with another negative feeling.

T: I feel like I kept it for a long time.

D: Now, still in that lifetime, go back to your mother. Is there anything you would like to say to her before you leave that lifetime?

T: No.

D: Scan your body. Are you holding onto any negativity caused by your mother in that lifetime? If so, allow it to come up your body and out of your mouth. It is time to release it.

T: (Long pause.) I guess that's where I get the sense that she doesn't love me because she didn't back then.

D: It is time to release the feelings that she doesn't love you. That was another lifetime, not this lifetime; you no longer need to hold onto it.

(I continued talking to her subconscious to release those feelings.)

T: (Gasps.)

D: Tell me what's going on.

T: I recognize the guy now! It's really strange; I don't know this person. He was a bartender at my mom's friend's party. But he was young and she was competing with me. I was young; it was really weird.

D: Give back to him any pain he caused you. Give it back to him. (Long pause.) Is it gone now?

T: Yes. I just left him there. (Becomes calmer.)

D: Tell me what's going on.

T: I'm dying.

D: Are there any lessons you learned from that lifetime that will help you in your current lifetime?

T: Life's too short. Follow your heart, but you can't make people love you.

D: Yes, those who are truly there for you will love you unconditionally. Are there any other lessons you learned from that lifetime?

T: Sometimes the people you trust, you can't, and sometimes the people you barely know will do their best not to let you down. There are no rules.

(We always have choices in life. I asked Tonya if she would like to see a glimpse into her future to view some of her choices. With her response being yes, the following came forth:)

T: I'm working. It's my own business and I know a lot of people.

D: How old are you?

T: Just – maybe a year from now.

D: Are you at peace?

T: I'm happy that I'm making my own money, and happy as a parent. I have a lot of friends, but there's something missing.

D: What is missing?

T: I won't let myself be in love.

D: Ask your subconscious. Is that to come in the future for you?

T: Yes, but I think I'm going to be angry about it.

D: Why is that?

T: Because it will be Johnny when he's ready, and when his wife leaves him and his daughter is old enough. And I'm just waiting.

D: Take a different direction into your future and allow it to unfold.

T: (Deep sigh.) I'm still working. It's the same thing, but not as hard. My daughter is confused and a little distant from me. There's a dark-haired man in my life, which is weird for me. He's very, very handsome and he has a job and he smiles a lot.

D: How do you feel about him?

T: I like him. But I feel like he's settling for what I can give him because I can't give him the love he wants or needs. I'm done. He's just there to waste my time.

D: What is confusing for your daughter?

T: She knows I'm in love with somebody else, and she really likes this guy. She can't understand why I can't be nice to him.

D: Ask your subconscious; is there a third road in your future?

T: Yeah.

D: If you are allowed to see it, allow it to come forward. Where does this third road take you?

T: Back to Texas. Nobody's happy about that.

D: How do you feel?

T: Desperate!

D: Why do you feel desperate?

T: Because I'm just following him, and I still don't have an identity of my own. But I just don't feel as sad because I'm next to him. But everybody else is mad at me. (Long pause.)

D: Tell me what's going on.

T: He leaves. His wife leaves. We end up together, but he feels like now I'm a responsibility because I went up there for him, and all I do is everything to please him. It feels like my first relationship. He didn't elect me to be there with him. I just went. I hate it there.

D: You see three crossroads; there is a possibility of a fourth. You have choices to make. Allow yourself to go deep within so you make the right choice in the future for yourself, for your happiness, for your highest good, the most positive choice for you.

T: Yes, there's another choice, but they won't let me see it now.

End of session.

"Wow, that was weird," Tonya said as she opened her eyes. "I loved him so much, I just didn't want to go on anymore."

As we discussed the session, Tonya finally understood her deep attraction and love for Johnny. He waited patiently for her in the past lifetime, then protected and took care of her, suddenly and violently dying at such an early age. She believed she could not go on without him, so thus took her own life at thirty. She was now rapidly approaching thirty again. Could this be why panic is setting in for her when he's not around, the fear of losing him again, yet their love relationship is not sanctioned because he is currently married to someone else? Timing? Is this karmic punishment for her for taking her own life in the past, or does it mean she now needs the patience Johnny displayed in the former lifetime? There were many questions and few answers, but at least there was the understanding about her uncontrollable love for Johnny along with some insight into her near future and the results of those choices.

Several months have past; Tonya has finally ended her romantic relationship with Johnny and recently met a wonderful young man. It is too early in the new relationship to determine the outcome, but I wish the best for her and her daughter.

Sally

Sally, a young woman in her early thirties, needed some answers. She appeared quiet and shy as she walked into my office. As we talked, she said she felt helpless and confused in her relationship with her boyfriend of several years. Her father was against their union and would not allow the young man to attend any family functions.

Sally had a history of migraine headaches, always beginning in her right temple, now occurring with more frequency. She had thorough medical checkups and an MRI with no signs of physical problems.

I regressed Sally back to the cause of her father's disapproval of her current life boyfriend.

It was the 1840s. She was Jennifer, a young brunette wearing a long blue dress with ruffles.

D: Look around. Where are you?

S: In a city.

D: Walk around. Describe the city as you are walking.

S: Brick buildings. The streets are cobblestone.

D: Continue walking. Go where you are headed. Where are you going?

S: I'm going to meet someone. I'm going to meet my lover, Alfred.

D: Look into his eyes. Feel his essence. Do you recognize him as someone in your current lifetime?

S: Yes. It's Louis, my boyfriend.

D: How did you feel about him in that lifetime?

S: I love him so much. We only meet in secret though, whenever we can.

D: Why do you meet in secret?
S: I don't think my father likes him.
D: Why doesn't your father like him?
S: He's not rich enough. He works hard, but he's not socially acceptable.
D: Move forward to a significant event in that lifetime.
S: I'm getting married.
D: The man you are to marry. Who is he?
S: It's the same person. It's Alfred.
D: How do you feel about the marriage?
S: I'm very happy.
D: How old are you now, when you are getting married?
S: I'm thirty-four.
D: Look around and see if you can find your parents. Are they there?
S: They are watching.
D: How do they feel about the marriage?
S: They're happy.
D: Why are they happy about Alfred now?
S: Because he's socially acceptable. He's very rich.
D: What type of work does Alfred do now?
S: He works for my father. He's really tall with a beard. He didn't used to have a beard before. My father likes him now.
D: What kind of work does your father do?
S: He's a banker.
D: Go to your house. What does it look like?
S: It's on top of a hill. It's two floors. It's really big with a lot of land. We're so happy now; we want to have some children soon.
D: Continue forward to a significant event. How old are you?
S: I'm thirty-six, (she replied quietly).
D: And how do you feel?
S: I'm very happy.

D: Where are you now?

S: I've gone to town to do some shopping; this isn't where I usually go, but I wanted to buy something special for my husband's birthday. It's getting dark. I forgot about the time. I must get back so Alfred doesn't worry. (She sits quietly for a minute, as though she's watching a movie.)

D: Tell me what is happening.

S: It's dusk. I decided to go down a cobblestone side street; it's a shortcut. (She begins fidgeting.)

D: What's happening?

S: I'm being followed. (She becomes more anxious.) I'm being watched. (Becomes more stressed.) No! No! They're coming after me! They've caught me!

D: Who are you referring to as they?

S: Two men. They've been watching me from the shadows. (Her chest begins heaving and she begins crying.) Oh, no! I shouldn't have gone down this road. I know better! (She begins sobbing.)

D: If your subconscious wishes you to view the scene as a movie, then allow yourself to do so. It is your choice.

(If the client begins showing signs of trauma such as deep breathing, sudden gasps of breath or facial changes, I offer the subconscious the choice of viewing the event as a movie, separating the client from the trauma or experiencing the event again.) Our subconscious is very powerful and knows what is best for the self. After the choice is made, the client continues with the unfolding of the lifetime. Chet Snow confirms this by stating:

A technique used by almost all of our therapists is one of becoming an observer. Patients seem immediately able to detach and observe unemotionally when the therapist gives permission for this. Often, a few moments of such objectivity make it possible for the patient to step back into the experience; supporting and not pressuring patients to actually re-experience overwhelming trauma but instead helping them to gain detachment from what they are experiencing until they are more able to deal with it.

S: (Her breathing became quieter and her body began to relax. Her subconscious decided it was too traumatic to relive the past experience.) They knocked me down and stole my jewelry and my money. I shouldn't have worn such nice jewelry. One man is hitting me on the head with a blunt object; I think it's a big stick. I'm bleeding – I can't move anymore. My dress is all dirty and ripped. (Sally is quiet again, as though watching a scene in front of her.)

D: What is happening now?

S: I see myself rising, but I also see my body lying on the ground. I think I'm dead. (Pause.) Yes, I'm dead – I didn't want to die.

D: Ask your Higher Self and subconscious if it is time to remove the pain caused by the severe blow to the temple.

S: (Long pause.) Yes.

(She was instructed to remove the pain, which she wanted to replace with peace.)

D: Your life was ended abruptly. Has this left a negative impact on that life, and if so, has this negative impact been carried over into your current life?

S: (Long pause.) Yes.

D: Ask your Higher Self and subconscious if it is time to remove this negative impact so that it will no longer hold you back in your current lifetime.

S: Yes, it's time.

D: Then allow it to be so. Allow yourself to remove all negativity from your abrupt and untimely death. Is it being removed?

S: Yes.

End of session.

~ ~ ~

After bringing Sally out of hypnosis, she stated that in her current lifetime, again her father didn't like Louis, the young man she has been dating, who was Alfred, her boyfriend and then husband in her former lifetime. Louis previously had dated her older sister, which is now causing much dissension among the family, so Sally has been seeing him in secret. The hypnosis allowed her to understand her love for this man in her life, reliving again her father's disapproval of him.

The regression also resolved many previously unanswered questions Sally had about her expensive taste. Ever since she was a young girl, she wanted only the most expensive, name-brand clothes and accessories. Her mother said even as a little girl, she would never settle for less than the best. At the time of the hypnosis session, she had been saving her money to buy a Gucci handbag, costing $1,025.00. Sally worked in a retail store as a salesperson, so her income was limited. I asked her why she didn't get a "knock-off" purse if that particular style was so important. She said, "No, I would never get an imitation. If I can't have the real thing, I won't have anything at all."

After contacting Sally over a year later, she said she no longer had migraine headaches, which prior to the session had been increasing as she was getting closer to the age the blow to the head occurred in her past lifetime. She has since changed jobs, as she says, "for the better." She is still with Louis, but he has not yet won her father's approval.

JOLINE

"It was instant," she said. "The moment Larry and I danced it was as though we had known each other for a very long time." Larry was Joline's fiancé and she was curious about their immediate and deep attraction. "He makes me laugh. I feel nothing can happen to me when I'm with him. He's my protector."

Joline was put into a deep hypnotic state. She was guided back into a past lifetime with her fiancé where she felt protected. She saw herself as a twenty-year old male named Bartholomew:

D: Tell me what is going on.

J: A book – books.

D: Feel the books. What type of books are they?

J: They're history. But they're not in English; they're in another language.

D: What language are they in?

J: Greek.

D: Why are all these books in front of you? What are you doing with them?

J: Researching, writing.

D: Look around. Is there anyone else around?

J: It's dark.

D: Why have you been left with the job of researching these books?

J: (Whispers.) I'm not supposed to be here.

D: Then why are you there?

J: Just curious – uncomfortable. I'm nervous; I'm not supposed to be there. It's like they don't want you to know.

D: Who are they?

J: The government.

D: How is it that you have access to the books?

J: My friend cleans there. It's night and he let me in.

D: Ask your friend to come forward. Is he there now?

J: Yes.

D: Look into his eyes. Feel his essence. Do you recognize him as someone in your current lifetime?

J: I'm not sure who it is.

D: It's okay. Move forward now to a significant event. Tell me what is going on.

J: (Gasps.) He gets in trouble for me being there!

D: Who found out you were there?

J: Guards. He's trying to explain that I was helping clean. (Takes deep breath.) It doesn't matter. I'm not supposed to be there. He's trying to take the blame for me. They don't care.

D: What is happening to your friend?

J: I got pushed out on the street and I never saw him again.

D: How is that making you feel?

J: (Takes deep, deep breath.) Guilty.

D: Scan your body. Are you holding onto that guilt in a part of your body?

J: (Grabs leg.) Lower part of my right leg hurts. (Begins fidgeting.)

D: Tell me what is going on.

J: It was Larry.

D: Is it time to release that guilt? You did something wrong and you tried to take the blame, but you were unable to. Is it time to release that guilt and the pain it is causing?

J: Yes.

(I guided her to release the guilt caused by that lifetime, filling the area with soft blue representing the power to move forward.)

D: What were the lessons you learned in that lifetime that can help you in your current lifetime?

J: Knowing when to stand up to authority. (Pause.) Trust. If he wanted, he could have turned the guards on me at any time.

> He trusted me not to say anything and I trusted him not to say anything. He protected me. He was there to help and protect. No, he was my best friend – he still is my best friend.

End of session.

Joline and Larry have a deep connection and trust that has been carried over into this lifetime. After the session, she understood the "instant knowing" she felt when she met Larry.

Many times clients under hypnosis recognize someone in their past life as someone in their current lifetime. This might indicate that many of us come into each lifetime together, playing different roles, here to help each other. When we help one another on the earth plane, there is the possibility we may find peace within.

Chapter 2

Healing Scars from the Past

How an event is perceived within the person can affect him positively or negatively down to the cellular level of his being. For example, as a young man Joe may have excelled in a sport in high school yet his parents, who had to take a second job to support the family, looked at the sport as a waste of time. In their minds, the time could be better spent in a job bringing in an income. This could cause mixed emotions for Joe: happy and excited that he did well in a sport he enjoyed, yet confused or even taking on guilt feelings over his parents' dismay. These feelings he may have internalized at a subconscious level could have a ripple effect to the point of sabotaging any future success. Finding the cause and understanding or removing the negative mindset can remove the blockage.

JANET

Events or people who come into our lives can trigger onset of pain. These energies are stored deep within our cells. Such is the case of Janet, a lovely woman in her forties. Her jaw began hurting seven months earlier and was getting progressively worse with a feeling of it "locking together." X-rays showed no fracture. A visit to the dentist confirmed no TMJ, a misalignment of the jaw, which can cause numerous problems from headaches to locking of the jaw. Within the past few days, she had a sensation of "bugs crawling in her throat." After putting her into a hypnotic state, we began:

D: Go to the original cause of your jaw feeling like it is locking together and bugs are crawling in your throat. (Pause.) Look at your feet; tell me what you see.

J: It's pieces of leather wrapped around the feet. It's like a cave. It's dark, and it doesn't smell good, and it's – it's a cave.

D: What does the smell bring up for you?

J: Like old animal fat, cooking.

D: Imagine looking up further. What are you wearing?

J: It's ratty looking, tattered clothing. It's just dirty. It's dirty in there, just unclean.

D: Are you male or female?

J: Female.

D: How old are you?

J: Early twenties.

D: Look around. Is there anyone around?

J: I don't see anyone. It's dark, I've got a light on a stick, and the end's on fire, like a torch.

D: What year is it?

J: I don't know.

D: Why are you in this cave?

J: It's like a tribe; it's where we live. It's what we have. It's all we have; it's shelter. It has other shadows, other openings to other – it's like dug out, underground, smooth. I felt like my jaw was "broke" earlier, it didn't want to move right.

D: Back up to just prior to your jaw being broken.

J: I was hit.

D: What were you hit by?

J: A man, just across the face. It broke my jaw.

D: Is he in front of you now?

J: Yes.

D: Do you recognize him as someone in your current lifetime?

J: I think it was someone – bushy hair, beard, and filthy. (Head jerks slightly, as though confused, then surprised.) It was someone I do know. That's someone who is a chiropractor.

D: Who is this in your past lifetime?

J: It's like a mate.

D: Now, go through the process of his hitting you. Did it break your jaw?

J: Yes.

D: Go into your jaw. Where are you holding onto the pain?

J: It's on the right side here. (Moves hand to side of face.)

D: What is causing the pain? What feelings are with the pain?

J: I didn't deserve to be hit. I didn't do anything wrong to be hit.

D: Go into your jaw. Imagine gathering up all the pain and begin throwing it back at him. He caused this pain. You did not deserve it. Scoop it up and throw it onto him. See it sticking onto him. And as you do, if there's anything you need to verbalize, allow yourself to do so as you throw it onto him. This is his problem; you no longer need to hold onto it. Give it back to him.

J: I don't want to get hit again! I don't want to be hit.

D: Tell him you're not going to be hit again.

J: I'm not going to be hit again! Take away the pain. Take your pain.

D: As you throw it back onto him, see it weighing him down.

J: He's walking away.

D: Have you gotten rid of it all?

J: (Nods her head yes.)

D: Now, see a balloon encircling the entire area with any remaining debris. If you were to give it a color, what color would it be?

J: Blue.

D: Imagine now, spitting this blue balloon out your mouth.

J: (Begins blowing and blowing for several seconds.) It's like something's crawling up the back of my throat.

D: What is crawling up the back of your throat? (Long pause.) You are in control. Find it!

J: It's like a bug.

D: What is causing this bug?

J: It's like an infection – rotten infection.

D: Go into the rotten infection. What is causing this rotten infection? Keep going to the cause of the infection. Keep bringing forth the cause.

J: It's my jaw. My jaw was broken, it was infected and I can't – I'm dying. (Keeps blowing air out of mouth.)

D: Keep spitting that rotten infection out. Have him in front of you and spit it out at him. You no longer need to hold onto that. Spit out the rotten infection, like a bug. Spit it out.

J: Begins coughing, almost choking, then begins blowing out again.) I'm dying. I know I'm dying! He doesn't want me here, so, fine. (Continues to blow air out of mouth.) I don't need to be with you then. I'm better than you. I'll be with you again! You've chosen that, I've chosen it. (Blows.) I'll be better off, and you know that I know that. I don't need this.

I never deserved this, but we had this. But you know what, it doesn't matter. He's forgiven; I just don't want to be with him. I just don't want this anymore.

D: Keep removing any leftover debris, until it's all gone.

J: (Coughs again, continues blowing.) This is the person I'm supposed to go to now for digestion. I just want to reach in and pull it out. (Takes her hand and appears to be pulling something out of her throat. Does this several times.)

D: Imagine now you have a hose with healing waters and it has a disinfectant in it. Allow it to wash throughout your body.

J: It's like a bubble of anger, just a last bubble. I know what it was! I was a healer and so was he, and I threatened him. (Whispers.) That shithead. (Blows again.) It's a bubble, and it's just working its way up. Come on; come on. I don't want to hold onto you anymore, you're not doing me any service. (Blows once more.)

D: Push it up and spit it out your mouth.

J: You owe me this lifetime to take care of me better. You know you do!

D: (Pause.) Are you completely cleansed?

J: Yes.

D: Ask your subconscious. Is he someone brought forth from your past into your present? Is he the one you need to go to, or is there someone else you need to go to for chiropractic healing?

J: No, he needs to do this! He has my tests.

D: Then allow your conscious to have all the information, so that you are aware of what has happened in the past and it does not transfer to your future.

J: It won't. There's still something right in the heart. It feels like something is stuck in my heart.

D: Go into the heart. Go to the cause of something feeling stuck in the heart.

J: (Long pause.) It was trust. He broke the trust. He broke it this time, too! (Blows air again.) You don't have to trust him. You can use him, but you don't have to trust him. You can empower yourself. You just need him for the tests, and you can take the test results elsewhere, you know that! But give him a chance to come up front. Get – (Blows again.) He's not as powerful – now it's coming. What is it you want me to know?

D: Go into what you need to know. Bring it forth. You can analyze it later.

J: Everything was a game! I don't play that. It wasn't to hold it back; it was to share it with others. Oh! (Whispers.) That's why you were pissed. (Speaks normal again.) It's not a game. The healing has to be shared with others. It's not for you to get rich, or to have things. You don't get it; you still don't get it. I'm here this time to remind him, (laughs), to share it with others. He doesn't have to get rich; that's not this purpose. He doesn't have to give it away either, but what he knows he needs to share and what I know, I need to share. All right. (Gets a strange look on her face.)

D: Is there more?

J: There's something working up. It's really deep. There's a really deep connection with this man. The circumstances were so bad. (Breathes heavily.)

D: Dig deep; allow it to keep working up.

J: It's like a bubble.

D: Allow yourself to be microscopic in size. Go to the bubble. And now, begin piercing that bubble, allowing the cause of the bubble to come forth.

J: I never really loved him; I just had to be with him. It was family; it was tribe; it was arranged. I didn't want to be with him and he knew that.

D: And this is what caused anger within him?

J: And it was jealousy. He was jealous of me.

D: Is there any more information in the bubble?

J: Something else wants to come out. (Whispers.) Come on. (Long pause.) He was such an unhappy man. He was very selfish. I irritated him. I was strong; it's almost like a starvation. He was very abusive toward me, but it still didn't stop me.

D: Keep bringing it forward. You have empowered yourself. You have brought back your power. It is time to release the bubble in your chest area. Bring it forward.

J: Oh! I wouldn't have children with him and I knew how to prevent it, and he knew I knew what I was doing, but he didn't know how. I shared that with other women. (Whispers.) Oh, that really pissed him off. (Blows air.)

D: See the bubble shrinking as you bring forth the information.

J: But I passed it on, and he couldn't do anything about it. See, he hoarded his and I didn't. I didn't want to be that important. I wanted to share what I knew, and he killed me because of it. I couldn't get to my stuff; I couldn't get to my herbs. (Speaking quietly.) But you know I have to let him go. (Keeps blowing air out of mouth.)

D: Has the bubble been released?

J: It's almost gone, but it's still there. I have to forgive myself for being submissive.

D: Are you ready to forgive yourself?

J: I loved myself even then.

D: Feel that love growing stronger and stronger. You were strong at that time, but he was physically stronger.

J: That's what the bubble is, and I forgive you because you couldn't cope with that. You didn't know how. We were in a time where male dominance – but I'll allow you to work that through now. You don't have to be dominant over me. There's no need. I won't allow it. Oh! You still want to be, but you're not going to be. (Continues to blow into the air.)

D: Is it completely over now?
J: It will be this week.
D: Then allow yourself to finish it properly.
J: Oh, it will be! It will be fine.
D: So there won't be any karma left.
J: There won't be. And he'll know.
D: Has the bubble been completely removed?
J: I think it's residual, but I think it will subside.
D: I ask your subconscious, will it completely subside this week?
J: Yes.
D: Then at that time, allow the skin of the bubble to weaken and be dissolved, the bubble to be removed.
J: Yes!
D: Allow yourself now to pass calmly, knowing you have removed all the pain, all the anger, looking up, going up to the light. See the light. (I continue guiding her to the light, having her pass through the light.) Is there any other time that has affected your throat or jaw area?
J: No.
End of session.

After the session, Janet said the chiropractor she was currently seeing, who was her mate in the past, had done several adjustments. During the third adjustment, as he was adjusting her legs, something "ripped on her side," causing great pain. She said she continued to go to him for two diagnostic tests that analyze fats, blood, etc. to understand which vitamins and minerals need to be added to enhance the proper functioning of her body. A week prior to her session, she became aware through her insurance company that the doctor was charging an excessive amount for his fees, over and above his previous quote. She said, "Part of him wants the best for others, the other part of him wants the money."

Since the hypnosis session, Janet said she is standing in her own power and has requested a transfer of her records to another doctor. She has been clear of all pain in her jaw and no longer has a "crawling" sensation in her throat.

SUZANNE

Suzanne was no stranger to hypnosis. We had worked together several years ago, and now she had an inner knowing that her life's path was changing. There were several issues she wanted to work on. First, Suzanne felt an urgency to connect with Buddha, her divine Grand Master and his healing energies. Second, would it be possible to see into her future to satisfy the inner feeling of pending changes in her life's path? And last, Suzanne said there are three women, she referred to as "ugly stepsisters," who are after her. Something intuitively told me to ask very little about the "ugly stepsisters," but let her subconscious under hypnosis bring forth what was troubling her.

You may find it interesting, as I did, when Suzanne was given permission to see into her future, she also brought forth information about Mother Earth.

After Suzanne went into a deep hypnotic state, she was taken back to the original cause of the "women after her, the ugly stepsisters." She saw herself as a twenty-three year old female named Aila, dressed in rags:

S: I stand there at the mouth of the cave. They want me to go into the cave and I don't want to go into the cave, but they're pushing me into the cave.

D: Allow the scene to move forward. Tell me what is going on.

S: (Long pause.) There's snakes in the cave, and they're going to throw burning light into the mouth of the cave behind me to drive me into the cave and to aggravate the snakes.

D: What was their relationship to you?

S: They're elders.

D: Are they male or female?

S: Female.

D: Ask them, why do they want to drive you into the cave and have the snakes come upon you?

S: I broke a rule. I used an herb that I wasn't supposed to use. I shared it with someone else, studying with him, telling how to use the herb.

D: What was the herb used for?

S: To travel.

D: What is the name of the herb?

S: It is called Geish. (Spelled as it sounded.) It would allow you to go on trips. It would be like the mushrooms now.

D: What year is this?

S: This was before they had time. It was a very ancient, primitive time. We were somewhere in Europe, when the stone places were used. This was a stone ceremonial place where the people worked with snakes.

D: Were the elders some of the people who worked with snakes?

S: They were associated. They served the men who did. I was not trained and they knew I would die. It was a sacrifice. (Appearing uncomfortable.)

D: Now, before we continue, if you wish to view it as a movie or go through it, it is your choice. Allow yourself to move forward and tell me what happens.

S: They were laughing at me.

D: How did that make you feel?

S: Shame and guilt.

D: Where are you holding onto that shame and guilt?

S: In my lower intestines.

D: Allow yourself to continue. Tell me what happens.

S: I didn't understand why they were so angry. I thought they taught me because I was to use these things, but only when they wanted me to, so I was afraid of the snakes. They were everywhere.

D: Where are you holding onto that fear of snakes now?

S: In my spleen.

D: Allow yourself to continue. Tell me what happens.

S: It took me a while to die from the poison.

D: What was associated with that poison?

S: I learned to use alchemy. It was the alchemy in the hallucinations. That was why I was able to travel. It was 300 years before Christ.

D: Allow yourself to scan that lifetime. Is there any other time within that lifetime you need to go to?

S: No.

D: What were the lessons you learned in that lifetime that will help you in your current lifetime?

S: No matter what happens, there's always good, there's always new information.

D: Are there any other lessons from that lifetime?

S: To forgive them.

D: Do you allow yourself to do so?

S: Yes.

D: Before we leave that lifetime, allow the knowledge of that lifetime to stay with you, so you do not bring the past into your future. You now have the knowledge. Is it now time to leave that lifetime?

S: Yes.

D: Imagine in your mind's eye looking up to the light and allow yourself to begin going to the light. Do you see the light?

S: Yes.

D: Imagine going up to the light, bringing with you only the positive from that lifetime. Now, allow yourself to go into the light, and as you go into the light, imagine burning up all the negativity as you continue going through the light. Allow the golden light to burn off all shame and guilt that was left over from that lifetime in your lower intestines. As you come to the area of the spleen, allow the golden light to continue burning all negativity so it falls away into ashes, falling away from you, cleansing the area of the spleen totally and completely from all fear of snakes that was put upon you in that lifetime. Allow yourself to continue through the light, intensifying the cleansing of the lower intestines and the spleen as you continue all the way through the light, taking with you all the positive aspects you gained from that lifetime, leaving completely and totally any and all negativity from that lifetime as though it was ashes floating down, allowing the ashes to fall onto the three elders. It is something you no longer need to hold onto; they caused it. As it falls on them, allow forgiveness to fall on them also. As ashes and forgiveness fall on them, allow their energies to be dissipated.

And now, going completely through the light, imagine yourself being re-born, renewed. As you go to the other side, imagine the dissipation of those negative energies rippling through each and every future lifetime up to your current lifetime, as though it were a rock thrown onto the water, having a rippling effect going out, each ripple affecting the next lifetime and the next, dissipating their energies completely and totally. Allow their energies to be removed from you, allowing you to become lighter physically, mentally, and spiritually. Imagine your energies glowing, a golden glow radiating from within, healing. Feel the healing taking place within. Now, imagine yourself in the universe, resting, at peace, energizing, gently floating back and forth, a new calmness taking over you. Any attachment you may have had from the past to the present has been cut away and the areas sealed so they no longer may reattach. Feel the lightness within, allowing your energy to grow stronger and stronger each and every day, a new awareness within.

As you are resting, growing stronger, allow yourself to connect with your divine Grand Master. Allow the energies to come forth, to be here with you. Feel the energies wrapping around you, allowing your Grand Master to be known to you. And now, allow yourself to tell me what is going on.

S: He's there, in a sage green, silvery brocade robe, silk. It is very delicate material. He's projecting energy around me.

D: Is there any information he wishes to bring forth for you?

S: He hands me a pomegranate. There are other beings here too, one on each side and one behind me.

D: And who are they?

S: Elohim. (Hebrew for God.) They are white. The pomegranate is full of seeds for me to ingest. It's like a power food that I always have with me. It is placed in my etheric stomach, just below my heart, that radiates a golden-red energy and vitality, divine vitality. As the seeds are needed, they will be released in my body for additional nourishment. There is an un-ending supply. This is a magic pomegranate. It's beautiful.

D: Is it beneficial for you to physically eat pomegranate?

S: Yes.

D: How often.

S: Whenever I need it. Whenever I want it. Whenever I need extra energy. But I don't have to actually drink or eat if I don't want to. It's there for my body to ingest in an etheric way.

D: You said there are three others, one on each side and one behind you. Who are they?

S: They're from the Elohim. They are angelic in nature. They are the angels that stay with the Supreme Being.

D: Do they have names for you?

S: No. They're part of a group. They're part of the golden-white light that comes from the Source. They are the embodiment of that light that travels as needed. Zoë brought them. His healing energies and his robe are also protecting me like a canopy around me. Like he wrapped his arms around me and I now wear that robe as well as the etheric pomegranate that is golden-red. It's like time-release medicine that is used today. It releases, as my body needs it. And we're done now. It is complete.

D: Thank you. You also mentioned Buddha. Is it necessary for him to be here today?

S: Elohim came from him. Not to worry, nothing to worry about. Just enjoy, be in joy, express joy. Happiness is the best medicine now, the only medicine that is needed.

D: Will you be allowed at this time to see into your future?

S: (Pause.) I am entering a school now, a new realm where I will travel in a new way, with less friction on my physical being. I am learning that now. The fear of going is removed. The distance that can be traveled is becoming greater. The work will become more specific in nature as to the tasks that are to be performed. Individuals will come that will need my help and I will be able to travel for them and release and remove obstacles.

D: While traveling for them, are you aware of the deeper meaning of this?

S: Yes, in between the worlds, into the unknown world, into spaces.

D: And in doing this, is there any additional information needed to protect yourself even further or are you completely protected now?

S: That has been given to me. The ring-pass-not (a golden ring of protection) has been enveloped around me. I will receive further instructions about this as time continues in school in preparation, as this work is unfolding now. The preparation, the schooling is unfolding now. I am entering a time of that preparation. This has been work today that has allowed me to enter that preparation at a higher level. Less time will be spent now in preparation because of the work done with the Elohim, Lao Tse, and the ring-pass-not, the ring of protection that has enveloped my body. It is a part of the new robe and the golden-red pomegranate. It is a source of food and nourishment when traveling to do the work to remove and shift energies, to release bondage, to clear and clean and elevate individuals so that they can be free to do their work, to be, to dream and create the new world. A time in birthing the Mother is completing. She is well through her birthing. That work is complete for me. It is not complete for her, but my time as mid-wife is done. She can come without my assistance. There are others working with her. I will shift into another level, preparing the others. Enough has been done with the Mother. A new task awaits me.

D: When you refer to the Mother, whom are you referring to?

S: Earth, Gaia, The Blessed Mother.

D: This need for added protection, this new level you are going to, are there others that you are aware of?

S: Others, many others. I will begin to know them as I shift into that task. Many others will still work with Mother. Many others are working in the etheric realm, preparing the place for the new earth, the place she is moving to and taking her children, the new world, the place of ascension, the place of elevated existence. It is a step, the next step, before the golden age can begin. It is a place of purification and manifestation and pure thought forms before we move into the golden age. All this is being prepared at many levels. I'm just changing from the level where we have been to where we will go in preparing that place. It would be like in your world today to build the nursery for the baby that is about to be born, to prepare a crib, a place to sleep and a place to be safe, with toys and fun and laughter, music to soothe the new baby, to care for the new baby, all the comforts for the baby. This is a time of joy in preparation for the new baby. That is the healing tool to be enjoyed and happiness and celebration for the birth of this new baby. The earth is the Mother and the baby. The old earth will die with the birth of the baby just like you celebrate the death of the old year and the birth of the new baby with the new year. It is like that.

D: As you move forward on your new path, are you able to identify others who will be working side by side with you?

S: There are so many. Just enlightened souls, evolving and growing. They walk the streets with you now, they drive cars, have homes. They have a higher purpose. They have moved away from greed and war and anger and work for a higher purpose, a higher source. They heard the call and are following their destiny, as we all will do in days to come. As the baby is birthed, many will join the ranks.

Many will go with the old earth and the old way and will recycle to be born again into a new place after they have been prepared, after they have gone to school and learned about the different time and the different needs and the different space that is available now. Some will go into the new place, the new earth, and not be quite prepared. They want to hang onto the old way, but they will be willing to learn and change. If they can learn and change they will stay. If they cannot learn and change, they will leave in the natural process called death in order to recycle, to return to school and learn again to be more prepared.

D: Is it allowed for you to see my path as we move forward into our future?

S: You are there, too. You are working in both places, both worlds now as this one is. Elizabeth is also there. There are many bright lights in the new place. Everyone is seen as a dot of white light. There are many. Some travel back and forth now and that's why they are so tired, because they work in both places at once.

D: Is this something that you and I are doing at this time?

S: Yes. Yes. You have seen the new place, the new space, the new nursery. If you were in a laboratory, there would be two petri dishes. One is old and one is new. One has dark veins running through it. That would be like mold or mildew to you, maybe. And so it has become corrupt. However, there is a new petri dish. It is filled with thousands, thousands and thousands of souls, white lights, like tiny pearls that are growing with luminescence. That is the new nursery. That is the new space. Some work in both places. Many work in both places to rescue as many as possible. There is choice, still choice, but that time is growing short, because the veins of dark and blackness have increased and gotten deeper and thicker in the old petri dish. It is becoming more and more unsafe to travel there, to rescue, and to bring back as many as possible into the birthing. There is a space between the two petri dishes. It is where the Mother is birthing, so this is the place where the snake sheds its skin and lets go of all the veins of the past, the dark veins that no longer serve mankind. There are those who will only be able to live in that petri dish. That petri dish will not be destroyed. It will become a school for those to learn about going to the next level, where there is light.

I'm looking at the two petri dishes, with the Mother in between the two, giving birth to those who would want to transcend, to let go of the old veins, to release their fear and their pain in order to move into the new. Those that are still working in the old petri dish take the pain into their body. This one is feeling that pain in the left kidney now. I've made many trips into the dark places to rescue.

D: Go into that kidney and give it a color. Surround the kidney with that color. You no longer need to hold onto that pain; it is time to remove the pain. What color is it?

S: Pink.

D: Surround the left kidney with the color pink. Begin pushing it down your leg onto the floor. (Pause.) Are you pushing it out?

S: Yes.

D: Continue pushing it out. Let me know when you are finished.

S: (Several deep breaths being released.) It's not going away.

D: Go into the cause. What is causing it to not be released?

S: Fear, of not enough people being saved, not enough people being found, not enough people being awake.

D: Allow your Master Guide to come forward and help you remove that fear. You no longer need to hold onto it.

S: It is not my responsibility to hang onto it. Enough work has been done. It's part of my responsibility here that I have not accomplished or achieved.

D: It is time to remove that fear. Ask your Master Guide to help remove it from you. You have been given high protection today, so you no longer need to hold onto that pain and that fear. Allow it to dissolve and flow down your leg onto the floor.

S: It's like a kidney stone.

D: Then imagine chipping away at it, breaking it up into tiny pieces.

S: (Pause.) It has dissolved.

D: Allow it to flow down your leg onto the floor, never to return. You have much work to do. You no longer need to hold onto fear. Has it been removed?

S: Yes.

(The area was cleansed and healed, filled with the color lavender representing peace.)

S: I'm surrounded by all the little white lights in the petri dish. There's really not much work to do there. The hard work has been in the old petri dish and at the side of the Mother. She has been birthing each one that has transformed and removed from one space to the other. She is tired, but smiles at me and thanks me. There are many working with her, too. They're strong, resilient. I took on too much there, fishing in the dark waters for those who were ready. It's time for me to stay in the new petri dish now.

D: Is it time now to leave, to move forward?

S: Yes.

(Took her to a peaceful place, again to rest and re-energize.) End of session.

I believe this session speaks for itself. Suzanne has been a healer for many years, and once she was cleared of ties to her past with the "elders," she was able to move forward into a new realm of healing others who come in contact with her.

Nancy

Nancy felt stymied in her job, as she described it, a "dead-end" career. This caused resentment and anger toward those around her for the slightest thing. It was time to get in touch with her anger. After hypnotizing her, we began:

D: Allow the information to come forth. What is causing the depth of the anger in your body? The anger deep within your body; allow it to come forward. Just take your time. Tell me what is going on.

N: It seems like ancient history, like Cinderella days, like knights. I don't know what century that is. I'm a female and I'm showing the side of my back, two men holding my arms.

D: Why are they holding your arms? What is the cause of them holding your arms?

N: They're holding me back from something.

D: Allow yourself to go forward just a small increment of time to a significant event. Why are they holding you back? What are they holding you back from?

N: They've got a man that they're taking away, and it feels like it's Jonah.

D: Who is Jonah?

N: My fiancé.

D: Is Jonah your fiancé in your current lifetime?

N: Yes.

D: Ask yourself, why are they taking him away? What is the cause of him being removed?

N: They don't want us to be here.

D: Who are they?

N: It's an evil man that is walking around laughing.

D: And who is this evil man? Does he have a name or a title?

N: Joseph.

D: What is his relationship to you?

N: I don't know. Something tells me that he's my brother.

D: Ask him, why does he want you two separated?

N: Because he's jealous, he's just evil, and he doesn't want to see anybody happy.

D: What is this causing in your body?

N: Anger!

D: Go into that anger. Where is that anger coming from within your body? Where are you holding onto that anger?

N: In my fists.

D: Go into your fists; hold onto your fists. Are there any other areas in your body that are bringing forth anger?

N: My chest and my throat.

D: Keep checking your body. Is there any other place that is causing anger within your body?

N: My forehead.

D: Imagine the anger in your forehead, chest, throat, and fists. Imagine it all being grouped into one lump. Now imagine grabbing it all and pushing it out your body and throwing it back onto this evil man, Joseph. Throw it onto him and as you do, also give it back to him verbally and physically. It is anger that he has put upon you. It is anger that has come from him that needs to be given back to him. What do you want to tell him as you are giving it back?

N: Just that what he says and does to me does not affect me.

D: Give it back to him. Allow it to come through your throat and your words. Give it back to him and allow this anger to stick onto him. You no longer need to hold onto it. He caused it.

N: He keeps laughing at me.

D: He can laugh all he wants, keep giving the anger back, and make the anger stick to him. Continue to release it from your body. Take it from your different body parts where it has been hanging on and give it to him.

N: (Deep sigh.) He's falling to the ground.

D: Keep throwing the anger onto him.

N: It's almost like – turning him blue and then pale. He's withering away.

D: Are you emptying the anger from all the parts of your body?

N: Yes, his body's disintegrating. It's in the ground.

D: Allow the anger to disintegrate with him, going into Mother Earth and being dissipated. Now, ask your body if there are any other areas that are holding onto anger caused by the man Joseph.

N: No. I'm finished.

(She was instructed to cleanse the areas with cool, clear, healing waters, and then wanted to fill the entire area with red roses representing love and empowerment.)

D: Allow your body to be filled with red roses, red roses of love and empowerment. Each and every time you see a red rose from now on, it will remind you of the love and empowerment within yourself. It will be a trigger that will bring forth that love and empowerment within you, growing stronger and stronger. Go back now to the time when the men were holding onto your arms. You have removed the anger and allowed yourself to be set free. Tell these two men who are holding onto you, you will no longer allow that to happen, you have set yourself free. Now, imagine freeing yourself. You are in control.

N: Yes. I'm free.

D: Go up to Jonah in that lifetime. What would you like to say to him?

N: We need to run away. (Deep breath, then releasing.) We're going toward my barn to get a horse, and we're going to get on the horse and ride away.

D: Allow yourself to do that; be free.

N: Away from the city and the negative world.

D: Are you riding off and away?

N: Yes, into a meadow where there are trees.

D: Allow yourself to rise above that lifetime and scan that lifetime. Is there any other time in that lifetime that your Higher Self or subconscious need to go to? If so, allow yourself to be there at a significant time.

N: I'm on my knees and I'm scrubbing the floors. It's still the same century. I'm a slave or peasant, whatever you call that. I don't feel like that's really what I am.

D: Is this still the same lifetime or is this a different lifetime that you've gone to?

N: I'm not sure.

D: Look around. Tell me where you are; describe what you see.

N: I'm in a house. It's more like a castle. I'm scrubbing the floors with a scrub brush.

D: Is there anyone else around?

N: Yes, there is a man sitting in a chair, almost like a king. I feel very out of place.

D: Ask your subconscious, your Higher Self, why do you feel out of place?

N: Because this isn't my potential, the life I really want. I don't want to be a slave.

D: Why is this a significant event within that lifetime?

N: Because it's making me angry.

D: Where are you holding on to that anger? Go to the cause of that anger in your body.

N: In my feet.

D: Ask your body and your subconscious, why is the anger in your feet?

N: Because I'm stomping. I'm stomping and swinging. I'm mad!

D: Who is causing you to be a slave and scrub the floors? Allow yourself to go to the person who is having you scrub the floors.

N: I've now stopped the scrubbing and I've run into the barn. It's at night, and there's a lantern, and there's lots of people outside, almost like they're going to a gathering. I hear them laughing at me because I ran to the barn. I go inside and I'm mad, but I'm not mad at anybody else. I just – I'm mad and I'm looking in the mirror. I'm mad at myself. I know I'm doing this to myself.

D: What are you seeing in the mirror when you look at it?

N: An ugly man.

D: Why is the man ugly?

N: It's my anger.

D: Where is the anger coming from?

N: Within me.

D: Go within yourself. Is this because, as you said earlier, you're not able to fulfill your full potential? Is that where the anger is being brought up from or is it anger from somewhere else?

N: I'm just angry. I don't really have a reason. I'm seeing and visualizing myself as a young mother looking into a mirror where there is an angry man, angry, ugly man. They're both angry. The faces are both angry.

D: Allow your subconscious and your Higher Self to bring forth the reasons for the anger, the reasons for the man and woman becoming one and the anger coming forward. Allow it to all come forth, bringing the anger within your body into words spewing out onto the mirror, releasing the anger as you do. Bring forth the cause that has been creating anger in this man and this woman.

N: (Pause, then deep breath.) I can see the man being chained up, almost like an animal. He's a big, heavy set, burly-looking man, but he's still really sweet inside, and they're beating him. The people are just stoning him and beating him – for no reason. I guess because he's ugly.

D: Who is this man?

N: I don't know.

D: Ask your subconscious, who is this man? Where is this man coming from?

N: Within me.

D: Allow him to come forward now. He is now in front of you and you are seeing him separate from your physical body. And now bring the woman forth, who is also angry. Allow her to come forth.

N: I'm angry at myself, and for some reason this beast or this ugly ogre-type man who I birthed – I birthed him.

D: This is an inner portion of yourself that you have birthed and brought forth? Is this what you are saying or is this inaccurate?

N: I don't know. I'm just feeling that this somehow, that this man is somehow tied to me through birth. Either he's my – it feels more like he's – I don't know.

D: Go over to this man and ask your subconscious, is this man a part deep within yourself that you have brought forth?

N: Yes, and I'm crying. I'm kneeling next to him and he's dying, and I'm crying.

D: Ask your subconscious, is it time for this ugly man within you, that is deep within you, is it time for him to die? He is a gentle soul. Is it time now to release the thoughts, the anger of being ugly?

N: Yes. All the ugliness around me is being shoved away; it's melting away. And now I can – I feel like when I'm holding him, he's a new person.

D: Then allow that ugly portion of him to die, holding him in your arms, allowing the sweetness and gentleness of him to stay alive within you.

N: I feel like I'm in heaven. He completely calmed my entire body. I almost feel like he created that monster to show me there is no monster. Everything's good, everything is on the surface. Fear, anger, that all went away.

D: Bless the ugliness that has been removed, because it was once a part of you. Bless it and allow it drain out your body onto the floor, to dissipate into Mother Earth. (Pause) Now, allow the birthing of the new you to come forth and go back into you, leaving the ugliness behind that you have blessed.

N: I'm holding a baby, like it's a new baby.

D: Allow the baby now to go in you, to become part of you. This is the new you, you have shed the old. Allow this new being, the beauty from within that has been separated from the ugliness of the man. Allow the beauty from within him that has become the baby to become part of you, to go in you, to be integrated within you. Feel the integration taking place, the birthing of a baby, a new you within. Have you integrated this baby within you?

N: Yes. I was holding the baby, then it shrunk down even further, and then I felt it go into me.

D: Allow it to grow stronger and stronger, the love and the beauty within yourself. And now allow yourself to be (Nancy interrupts.)

N: I have a little boy holding my hand, and he's tugging on my hand! We're in the zoo, we're in an underground part of the zoo with the animals, and I feel like this little boy's in myself. I don't know, I just feel happiness, happiness all around us. He's happy and I'm happy. He's making me so happy. (Begins crying.) He's – and he's smiling, and he's pointing and laughing. He's making me happy. (Continues to cry.)

D: Ask your subconscious and your Higher Self, who is this little boy representative of?

N: The son I'm going to have.

D: Is there any more information?

N: (Shakes head no.)

D: Allow it to just be. Enjoy it for another moment. You will know him when he comes forth. He is waiting for the right time to come forth. Is there anything else he wants to tell you before he leaves?

N: He's says it's going to be okay mommy. He's massaging my head. (Still crying.) And he's waving at me goodbye – and he's going back.

D: Ask your subconscious and your Higher Self; is there anything else you need to address at this time that is causing any pain or any anger within your body?

N: I don't feel any anger.

End of session.

Nancy had separated from herself. This was indicated when she said, "I'm visualizing myself as a young mother looking into a mirror where there is an angry man, angry, ugly man. They are both angry. The faces are both angry." The ugly man was created by the anger within her. Once removed, the inner child or new birth came forward and was integrated within her. She was no longer consumed by anger toward herself and others. A calmness came over her, and with that an unexpected caring and renewed love for herself.

Elena

Elena was in her mid-thirties, working in a comfortable job for a tax broker. She had her CPA degree, but was afraid to take the next step and start her own company, which would give her more independence. She was complaining about the fear of financial success. "Why does it elude me?" she said. "I come so close, then something inside says I really don't want to be successful. Why does this keep happening? I'm tired of this; I want to be my own boss."

After the hypnotic induction, Elena went back to the cause of her fear of financial success. She saw herself as Sam, a man with dark hair in his mid-thirties, wearing a suit, "like a zoot suit."

D: Tell me where you are. What do you see as you look around?

E: It's an office. There are some desks. There's some money on the desk.

D: What is your job at the office?

E: I think I'm the manager. I'm in charge of the money.

D: What type of office is it?

E: Banking.

D: Does this banking firm have a name?

E: Looks like Bank of America.

D: Tell me what's going on, in detail.

E: It's the market crash! It's the market crash. I had something to do with losing lots of money. (Pause.) I committed suicide! I committed suicide.

D: Allow yourself to go with that. Tell me what is going on.

E: There's a lot of chaos and there's a lot of stress.

D: Go into that stress.

E: It's in my neck and my chest, my stomach.

D: Gather it all together and allow it to come forward. Verbalize the stress.

E: The stress is from loss of lots and lots of money, everybody's savings. It's not just mine, it's everybody's savings. It's gone. People are praying. I hurt in my chest. I'm responsible.

D: Go to the time prior to your death.

E: I'm still alive, and I'm just feeling horrible. I feel bad that I lost all this money. It's not mine – people's life savings. I'm crying. People are screaming.

D: Is it time to remove this pain in your chest caused by the market crash? You are not the cause of the loss of the investments because of the market's crash.

E: But people think I was responsible!

D: You have held onto this pain long enough. It is time; allow yourself to begin removing the pain from your chest.

E: (Deep breath.) My chest is clearing out now. (Again she takes a deep breath, blowing air out.) It feels lighter. I'm not responsible. People think I was, but I'm not. This is just something that happened.

D: Keep removing the pain.

E: It's in my head, too. I'm clearing the head. My head's clearing, my poor head. Oh! That's where I landed when I jumped. It was a lot of pain. I'm in my pajamas – all that tension. I'm not responsible.

D: Keep pushing out that tension and stress. Remove that sense of responsibility. You no longer need to hold onto it. It was not your choice to have the market crash.

E: I'm releasing the peoples' energies I feel responsible for, too.

D: Keep releasing it. It may be one at a time or in groups. They may have faces or be faceless. It is your choice; just continue to remove it.

E: They're just staring at me!

D: Continue to release their energies from your body.

E: (Long pause.) I'm letting a lot of energy out, but it's not mine. It's everybody's energy. I don't need their energy. I'm strong and powerful myself. I take on everybody's energy thinking that they'll give me strength, and they don't give me strength. I'm releasing everybody's energy from my face. I'm going down my leg to release. My right leg, there's something wrong there. There's something there. Okay, I feel a lot lighter; I feel much better.

(She is currently a Reiki Master, so I incorporated this into the hypnosis.)

D: Take your right hand and put it behind your neck, and heal any remnants from the problems from your neck, arthritis, any negative energy. Feel the Reiki energy going through your neck, healing your neck. You have powerful energies. As you are healing the back of your neck, feel the powerful healing energies coming forth, healing the front parts of your neck. Feel it now flowing down your body, healing your body.

E: My shoulders, too. I'm taking back my power, too. It's interesting, my power in my neck and my shoulders are not connected. The light's so bright. I don't even know what it is; I'm just releasing it.

D: Ask your subconscious, do you need to know what it is in order to release it?

E: Yes.

D: Go into the remains of what is holding on. Bring forward the cause.

E: I keep getting this horse thing.

D: Bring forward the cause of the leftover pain in your neck.

E: I've got a yoke on.

D: Go into the yoke. What is the yoke bringing up for you?

E: Just tired and worn out, not wanting to have this yoke on. It's a horse's yoke, but it's a person's yoke, too! Oh! I'm a person way back. The yoke, I'm carrying two buckets of water, sandals on my feet. I just had to carry this water all the time. I was a water bearer. I'm just tired.

D: Is it time to release that stress from your neck?

E: Yes.

D: Feel it leaving your neck. Allow it to dissipate.

E: I'm just tired, it's just tiredness. I need to let the tiredness go. It's not pain, it's just tiredness.

D: You may now release it. Release the energies of being tired from that lifetime. Make a small hole if you wish, letting the air of tiredness out to be released.

E: I'm making a big hole!

D: Release all the feeling of being tired and worn out from that hole.

E: (Deep sigh.) That feels good. It's going all the way down on my spine.

D: Keep releasing it, removing it from your spine, letting it out from that hole.

E: It's almost gone. It's leaving my hips now, and my head now. I'm feeling lightness. (Pause.) I feel something in my throat.

D: Go into the throat area.

E: It's tingling.

D: Go into the tingling. What is causing the tingling?

E: My whole face is distorted.

D: Go into the distortion. Bring it forward.

E: It's a disease. It's like a disease that's all over my face and my neck. It's just like I had this horrible look. I was a man. I'm releasing it; it's no longer mine. I had it for a long time. I had ridicule and embarrassment. I'm releasing the feeling of not wanting people to look at me, that I'm not okay, that I'm horrid. I released that. (Begins moving in chair.)

D: What else is there?

E: Fear. People would attack me because I looked ugly – throwing rocks. This was a long time ago when they didn't understand it. Releasing it from my eye, being ridiculed, not being able to say or express all this hurt, and being sad that nobody would want me because I was so distorted. (Pause.) Epileptic comes through, leprosy. Nobody wanted me. I can feel the leprosy.

D: Is it time to cleanse your body?

E: (Long pause.) I've got the face done. Oh, that was a tough one! Releasing that ugly face, and I have a beautiful face now. It was mostly my face, and now my body. I'm almost whole. It feels good. (Pause.) I've got something else again. Another lifetime is coming in, pain in my neck!

D: Bring the cause forward. Go deep within the neck area. Go into the cause of the pain in your neck.

E: I think I was cut. I was stabbed.

D: What is causing the cut, the stab in your neck?

E: I want to put a golden light over it. There's a lot of crying. It's sad. I'm not wanting to speak. Oh, I just embarrass myself when I speak. Whatever I say, it just doesn't come out right. It's like my mind doesn't formulate right. When I say something, it comes out funny. I go so fast that I'm ahead of myself and people don't know where I'm at.

D: Become microscopic, walk around in the brain; check the brain. See if there is any loose wiring.

E: It's on the side of my head.

D: Test all the wiring within your brain. Rewire if necessary.

E: I'm straightening everything out. It's clearing now. It's been a long time since I could really talk. I'm saying the words correctly so people can understand me. I'm not jumping around. I can slow down now.

End of session.

Elena now understood her hesitation on starting her own business. She was still dealing with other people's money, only in a different way. She was now ready to "start on her own." She had been having dull headaches more recently, but "didn't think much about it." There is the likelihood that her headaches were caused by her falling on her head when she committed suicide, recurring as she neared the age she was when the incident occurred in her past life.

Some patterns in the current lifetime originate in past-life traumas, where the subconscious is trying to uncover and resolve issues hidden below the surface. These patterns help to understand the dynamics of existing problems and situations and allow the client to see the roots of certain choices in everyday life. He becomes aware of associations and receives insights to help his growth. These can be released or reframed, depending on the subconscious' desires. The traumatic event, brought into the consciousness, often creates a cathartic release and removal of previous negative symptoms. Understanding our behavior and feelings from other lifetimes allows forgiveness, which in turn may release the guilt we put upon ourselves.

"People have the idea that free will and destiny are opposing forces," according to Dr. Michael Newton, author of the book, *Destiny of Souls: New Case Studies of Life Between Lives*. He states:

> They do not realize that destiny represents the sum of our deeds over thousands of years in a multitude of incarnations. In all these lives we had freedom of choice. Our current life represents all past experiences both pleasant and unpleasant, and so we are the product of all our former choices. Add to this the fact that we may have deliberately placed ourselves in situations that test how we will react to events in our current life, which are not perceived by the conscious mind. This too involves personal choices.

During a follow-up call to Elena, she said that her headaches have ceased and her energy has increased. She doesn't feel "weighed down anymore."

Energy blocks may be caused from several lifetimes, not just one. In the case of Elena, her subconscious jumped into several lifetimes to remove obstructions.

SANDY

A gifted psychic, Sandy began questioning her abilities and the information coming forth. She said, "I've been given this beautiful 'gift of sight,' but I have a fear growing inside associated with it that I don't understand."

Inducing a hypnotic state, Sandy was taken back to the cause of her fear of her "gift of sight."

D: Look around. Where are you?

S: In China.

D: Allow China to come into focus. Look at your feet.

S: I'm a man, with little black shoes, brocade robe, a silk robe, and little black hat.

D: How old are you?

S: I am in my early thirties.

D: What is your name? Why are you there?

S: I am a seer, that's what I am. My name is ShiQuan.

D: Look around. Tell me what you see.

S: The Emperor is angry. His wife is afraid. There are things I've had to say that are upsetting. They cannot stop the army that will kill him. There's no way I can stop the army. I am going to be banished. He is going to send me to stop the army.

D: Allow the scene to unfold. What are you doing?

S: I am drinking the poison. I don't want to die there. They are barbarians.

D: What year is it?

S: 1650.

D: After you drink the poison, tell me what happens.

S: He is infuriated, so my body is disposed of in a disgraceful way – to disgrace me.

D: Go back to the time when you drink the poison. What is it causing in your physical form?

S: Great pain.

D: Where is this pain in your body?

S: In my stomach.

D: You were disgraced because you had a great gift of sight. The Emperor did not understand; he did not wish to understand. Is it time now to remove the pain that was caused from drinking the poison?

S: (Nods yes.)

(I instructed her to remove the pain caused by drinking the poison and cleanse it with healing water. She replaced the area with gold, silver, and white light – to her representing the highest white light.)

D: Is your body holding on to any of the disgrace when the Emperor disposed of your body in a disgraceful way?

S: There was some in my spleen, but it's moving.

D: Where is it moving to?

S: It's in my left ovary.

D: Is there any other area besides your spleen and ovary?

S: No.

(I instructed her to have cool, clear water, spraying into the spleen, flowing down into her ovary, cleansing and healing the entire area.)

S: It's clean.

D: Scan your body. Are there any remnants left over from that lifetime, any fear, being afraid of your gifts of sight?

S: There's some poison still left, right here. (Points to side.)

(She was instructed to cleanse the area and fill it with white light.)

D: Are there any other areas that you need to go to within your body?

S: No. I'm finished.

D: Scan that lifetime. What were the lessons you learned from that lifetime?

S: Not everyone wants to hear what you have to say. Sometimes what you have to say is dark. It's not wise to take your life, other events could have happened. Don't give up in despair, there's always hope.

D: Are there any other times in your past lives where you are holding onto pain caused by your gifts of sight?

S: (Long pause.) I'm a peasant, and I'm dirty.

D: Why are you dirty?

S: There's mud all over me. I've been thrown into the mud.

D: Are you male or female?

S: I'm a female.

D: How old are you?

S: Seventeen.

D: Why were you thrown into the mud?

S: I'm a heretic. I can't behave myself. I can't keep my mouth shut.

D: What are some of the things that you say?

S: I'm in disagreement with the church. The man won't let me in the house.

D: Who is the man to you?

S: He's the elder, the authority. Fighting with him won't do me no good, and I've already crossed the threshold with him. I can't go back. All the doors in the village are closed.

D: Go to the next significant event. Tell me what is going on, in detail.

S: I'm cold, wet, hungry, freezing. I'm dying of the cold.

D: What year is it?

S: 1453.

D: What is your name?

S: Elsa.

D: Just before passing over and dying, tell me what is going on.

S: I'm crying. I wonder why I can't fit in, why I can't accept, why I can't go with the flow.

D: Why were you given this gift in that lifetime?

S: Choices are just choices. It doesn't matter; it doesn't matter. (Pause.) It's better to be in your truth than to negate who you are and what you know. Discernment is the lesson.

D: Where are you in your truth in that lifetime?

S: My truth got me thrown in the mud – thrown out.

D: But you were in your truth, what you came in that lifetime to do.

S: (Deep sigh.) Yes. I could have also chosen to be wise and silent and watch the outcome, however it was not my choice and that was okay.

D: Now that you know that it was okay to speak out the truth, the gift of your sight, is it now time to remove the suffering from that lifetime because of the gift of sight?

S: Yes.

D: Is there any specific area within your physical form that is holding on to that pain?

S: It's in my neck, my side.

(I instructed her to remove the pain from her neck and side. Next, she wanted to fill the area with a light turquoise color representing joy. Took her to the light to cross over.)

Since this was a traumatic past lifetime, at the time of her death I instructed her to look up and go "to and through the light." This is to imagine cleansing and leaving behind any negativity caused by that lifetime, bringing forth only the positive insight gained.
End of session.

Sandy said she felt a heavy load had been lifted from her body. She was different as a child, being teased by other children, told "not to speak of such things" by her parents. She said her abilities seemed to disappear, only to come back in her mid-thirties. She finally understands the fear she has held on to for many years in speaking her truths. She is now comfortable with herself and the beautiful gift she was given.

Chapter 3

Chronic Pain

It is extremely important to obtain good medical advice and treatment of any injury or disease we suffer. After taking care of the problem with proper medical help and treatment, if a pain still lingers for no apparent reason it can cause other problems such as emotional depression or in time physically affecting the heart, kidneys, liver, colon, or even blood pressure.

When chronic pain begins to affect a person's daily life, it's time to take steps to improve the quality of that life and remove the pain. The patient's lack of belief in hypnosis has little to do with his benefiting from it. Hypnosis does not involve drugs or needles, yet it is so powerful that surgeries, dental extractions and the delivery of newborns have been done with hypnosis as the only anesthetic.

EVELYN

Evelyn complained of chronic pain in her left hip. She has been seeing a chiropractor for several years. Her left leg was constantly "going out," causing her spinal misalignment. When the leg was "out," her left leg was shorter than her right, causing her to walk with a limp. X-rays showed no degeneration or weakness in the area, but she said, "The leg just would not stay in place."

After Evelyn was hypnotized, she was taken back to the cause of the pain in her left hip.

D: Where are you?

E: Egypt, the temple.

D: What are you doing in a temple?

E: We're moving stones.

D: Who are we?

E: Me and my brothers – not slaves, we volunteered. Need to make money for family, to protect them, provide for them. So thirsty, weak, just want water.

D: What are you doing now?

E: Pulling a stone, high on the temple. Need water – no!

D: Tell me what is happening!

E: He's whipping me.

D: Who's whipping you?

E: The guard. I just wanted water. So thirsty – lost my balance, I didn't let go of the rope when I fell. Oh, there's so much pain!

D: What is causing the pain?

E: The stone came down on me, cut my leg off, crushed, pulled it away.

D: Scan your body. Where are you holding onto the physical pain?

E: In my hip.

D: Go into your hip. Ask your subconscious, is it now time to remove the pain from your hip caused by it being severed from your body? (Evelyn begins to fidget in her chair.) Tell me what is going on.

E: Where is my leg? I can't find my leg!

D: Do you need to find your leg in order to remove the pain?

E: Where is my leg?

D: Find your leg. What happened to your leg?

E: My body is just lying there. Nobody cares. Everybody's just going about their work, they don't care. People die all the time. They just pulled my body away; it was there for days.

D: Find your leg. What happened to your leg?

E: (Long pause, then a deep sigh.) Oh, it's part of the temple. My leg is sealed in the temple. It's part of the mortar; it's in a sacred place. My family hates me; my brothers hate me.

D: Why does your family hate you?

E: Because I left them. I can't work anymore.

D: It was not your fault that you died. You were working to help support your family. You were doing the right thing trying to support your family. Go to your family. Is your family there?

E: Yes.

D: Ask them if they hate you.

E: No, they don't hate me, they're crying because I'm gone.

D: Go to your brothers. Why do you think your brothers hate you?

E: Because I left them. My brother got me the job; it was a good job; I made money.

D: Ask your brothers if they hate you for leaving. It was not your fault that you died.

E: They're here. They're sorrowful, sad that I'm gone. I was wrong.

D: Now that you have found your leg, is it time to remove the pain?

E: Yes.

D: Go into the hip area and begin pushing out the chronic pain that you have been holding onto for so long, caused by your leg being severed from your body in that lifetime. Feel the hip area being healed. Feel the healing energies taking place. (Pause.) Is the pain completely removed from the hip?

E: It's leaving. I still have a little left.

D: Keep removing it.

E: It's almost gone.

D: Take your time. Remove it completely.

(Evelyn then wanted the area to be filled with the color pink, representing love.)

End of session.

In discussion after the session, Evelyn said her body lay there for several days. "Nobody said any prayers over me, which was really sad. Then somebody came with a cart and picked up my body with others that had died or been injured. It was days before anybody picked me up. It really hurt my feelings."

Dr. Francesca Rossetti, author of *Psycho Regression: A New System for Healing & Personal Growth*, states:

> Everything on earth is made up of energy, vibrating at different frequencies, depending upon the atomic structural pattern within the atoms and molecules. When these energies are disturbed they become stuck or clogged up like a drain, the energies remain static until they are finally able to loosen and reform themselves harmoniously. The same thing occurs within an individual's unresolved karmic energies. Like an orchestra we are comprised of many parts, each instrument working harmoniously together in order to create the best possible sound.

~ ~ ~

A week later, Evelyn called to thank me. She said she went to the chiropractor the next day and he said, "What's the matter, it's not out, it's back where it's supposed to be." She continued, "Usually when I go in to have him fix me, one leg would be much shorter than the other, but nope, everything's fine. They were the same length, because when it would go out, one leg would be longer than the other, then when you try to walk, it affects your spine all the way up."

The hypnosis session was several years ago. In a recent conversation with Evelyn, she said, "I haven't been back to the chiropractor, and I haven't had any pain or discomfort in my hip since then."

I believe Evelyn's pain in her hip was negative energy that had never been released at the cellular level. It was partly caused by the leg being severed at the hip from her body, but also caused by her not knowing what had happened to the leg and a belief that her family "hated" her.

ESTHER

Complaining about pain in her shoulder, Esther decided to try hypnosis. The doctors could find nothing, but the dull ache in her shoulder and sometimes in her neck had been with her for some time now.

Once in a hypnotic state, Esther was taken back to the cause of pain in her neck and shoulder:

D: Where are you?

E: I'm outside.

D: What are you doing outside?

E: We're standing.

D: When you speak of we, whom are you referring to?

E: My people. You are there; Thomas is there. (Smiles.) Spiritual teachers. (Begins to frown.) A messenger had come and said they were coming for us. We prayed about it and decided to meet them outside so they wouldn't tear up the community and talk to them. They're lining us up.

D: Who is lining you up?

E: The soldiers.

D: What kind of soldiers are they?

E: Romans.

D: Why are the Roman soldiers lining you up?

E: No! They're slaughtering everyone!

D: Why are they slaughtering everyone?

E: Because of our beliefs.

D: And what are your beliefs?

E: They're treating us like criminals. (Deep sigh.) They're getting slaughtered, all the women and children.

D: Why are they slaughtering just the women and children?

E: It's not just the women, the children; it's all of us. Other people had their children standing with them, and the soldiers came; they didn't slow down at all. (Begins squirming.) The children were out in front, and they ran right over the children, just trampled them.

D: What is the time frame, the year?

E: I don't know. It's before the Messiah.

D: What is your name?

E: Ruth.

D: Allow yourself to move forward to a significant event.

E: (Long pause.) They just slaughtered them. It's a blade, went in my back.

D: Are your children with you?

E: No, they're hiding. I didn't want them to hurt the little children. I just didn't want to take the chance, so I sent them out. Some of us sent them out. I was confused, I was really afraid. I was scolded because I sent them out, up into the mountains to hide. They're sending soldiers everywhere. Be prepared – ooohhh, there's so much pain. They killed the children. (Deep sigh.) I'm bleeding.

D: What has happened?

E: (Takes a deep breath, lets it out.) I'm kneeling. Not a very big woman, just a little thing. I'm praying. A soldier came up to me and took his sword, put it through me. It went through my shoulder, through the top of my leg. – ooohhh, through the back of my leg. (Wrenches.) He pulled it out. (Deep sigh.) I'm bleeding. He just stabbed all these people; we were just massacred; we never tried to fight.

D: Go into the area you are bleeding from. Ask your Higher Self, is it time to remove the pain caused by the sword going through you in that lifetime, from your current body?

E: I just want to remember.

D: What do you want to remember?

E: The good things we were doing.

D: Then allow the good things to come forward and verbalize them.

E: We were teaching everybody about the Messiah's coming, the church, and what's going on with them. We taught people to share in the divine grace. We taught honesty, understanding, compassion, although we were not always compassionate. We kept records. We were born to prepare the way for the birth of Christ, the Messiah.

D: Where are the records?

E: The children, we gave them to the children to hide. We kept scrolls, and they were to take them into the mountains and hide along with the scrolls in the caves.

D: Are the records hidden?

E: Yes.

D: Is there any more positive information to bring forth at this time for your remembrance?

E: (Deep sigh.) No one resisted. Nobody raised a hand. Nobody shouted. Nobody screamed and ran.

D: Why did no one resist?

E: It was our choice. It was our teachings.

D: Is it now time to remove the pain caused by the sword and the pain from that lifetime?

E: Yes.

(Went through the process of removing the pain.)

D: Scan that lifetime. What were the lessons you learned from that lifetime?

E: It was more important how we died than how we lived. It was the dignity that was shown in our deaths, not the way we lived, not the Essene gospels that were protected. How we died showed them the kindness and the respect that the community deserved. It changed them; it touched their lives. That was the whole purpose. Many of the soldiers who fought and killed in that battle later became Christians and turned against the Roman government. We don't come back often; we come back in the time to do battle.

End of session.

In discussion after the session was over, Esther said it was one of many Essene communities. She said it was a beautiful village. "We showed them that we weren't a violent cult to be afraid of. We never fought back; we never raised a hand to them. Our accomplishment was in how we died, not so much how we lived. I always had this place in my neck and shoulder that hurt me really bad. Now I know it's because when he pulled it out, it nicked across the side of my head, and then he just went wack!"

Chronic physical pain may stem from traumatic injuries or deaths incurred in past lives, especially trauma to the head, limbs, and the back. Going back to the original cause often releases or reduces the pain in these areas.

I am adding her further comments about that lifetime, as I found it interesting. Esther continued, "Everything had become corrupt, so we moved away and started our own village - everybody for one. It was a good life when I was living in the city before, but then my husband and my family, the men, were not happy with what was going on in the temples. They were charging us to go pray, because someone came up with the idea to make more money. Everything had a price. We decided to move because not everything had a price. There was no price on our soul. It was a good life because even though we were all killed, something was accomplished. These men who took our lives all changed."

In contacting Esther years later about the pain in her shoulder and neck area, she said, "the pain has never returned." As with Evelyn, I believe the pain in Esther's neck and shoulder was caused by negative energy that was carried into this lifetime at a cellular level. Once she was able to understand the cause of her pain, she was then ready to subconsciously remove it.

HENRY

Several years ago Henry entered my office. I was surprised when he said he was in his mid-sixties, as he appeared much younger. He said, I "was his birthday gift." His girlfriend thought it would be a new experience for him and paid for my services. He didn't believe he could be hypnotized nor did he believe in past lives. Henry asked to be taken back into a past life, wanted dates and facts so he could research the information later. Part was his curiosity and part was to prove to himself and his girlfriend that hypnosis and past lives were all a "hoax."

So many of my clients, when they go back to the "cause" of their deep-rooted issues, go back to past lives where their issues began. This is brought forth into their current life in the form of emotional or physical pain or suffering. Because of this I am a believer in past lives. Although this is my belief, I have never forced it upon anyone else. A belief in past lives is not necessary to release unresolved trauma that does not stem from childhood. Many clients do not believe in a past life or have questioned the theory. When this is the case, prior to hypnosis I tell the client that the subconscious may create a story or a fantasy in order to release whatever is necessary. This does not in any way interfere with removing negative energy blocks.

Even though Henry didn't believe he could be hypnotized, he complained about a pain he had in his right shoulder for the past fifteen years. He described it as a dull ache, but it was something he "learned to live with." He had been to several doctors over the years but they could find nothing wrong.

I regressed Henry back in time to a prior lifetime. He went back to the time of the civil war and saw several people he recognized as friends in his current lifetime. This brought emotional tears to his eyes that surprised him. When he had sufficient names, dates, places, and descriptions of clothing apparel from that time period, I guided him to the light, cleansing his physical and spiritual self from all negativity from that lifetime and bringing forth only the positive and any knowledge gained from that lifetime.

While he was still hypnotized, I asked Henry if he would like to go back to the cause of the pain in his shoulder. He said, "no." I decided to take another approach to his firm statement of "no." I had not been faced with a client not wanting to remove pain before, so I decided to ask his subconscious and Higher Self if permission would be given to remove the pain without going back to the actual time the pain was caused. He immediately responded, "yes." I asked him to imagine shrinking himself to a microscopic size and going into his physical form in the area of the pain in his shoulder. This microscopic version of him was equipped with a magic toolbox, with any tool he wished at his disposal. It could even be a tool of his own creation. He was then instructed to walk around and find a dark mass creating the energy block. Once he found it, he began chipping away with his creation of a power drill used for breaking up cement. After he broke up the entire mass, he poured a special dissolving solution on it, melting the mass. Then he was instructed to allow the liquid mass to drain down his arm and out his fingers through the openings at the end of his fingers. He cleansed the area using a hose with magical healing water. He then sprayed a sealant around the shoulder so the mass would not form again and filled the area with the color blue that to him represented strength in his shoulder.

When Henry came out of hypnosis, he was surprised and elated that his civil war experience was "so real." He was going home and immediately checking the validity of his information gained on names, dates, and places.

He became quiet for a moment and softly told me even though he did not want to go back to the cause of the pain in his shoulder, he knew what had happened. He saw himself as a foot soldier in the middle of a battle in the 1400s. An enemy on horseback charged up to him and with one fell swoop of the sword cut off his right arm at the shoulder. It is my belief that with the excruciating pain and the possibility of his surviving for a period of time before dying, the suffering and agony that was caused left a tremendous amount of blocked energy within that area, which he brought into his current lifetime.

Henry called me several months later to say he had complete mobility in his shoulder and has not had pain since the hypnosis session. He has now been free of shoulder pain for several years. Although his civil war dates and some details were not exact, he was satisfied that the information was "close enough."

Chapter 4

Healing Our Wounded Spirit

Back into His Arms

When something traumatic happens to a person his spirit or inner self is wounded. The event may be so traumatic that he stores it in his subconscious, yet does not remember the trauma consciously. This trauma may have occurred as a small child. Now he is an adult, and certain events not related to the trauma may trigger the unresolved hurt feelings and emotions. In order for healing to take place in the wounded spirit, he needs to go within himself, back to the age the original trauma occurred, and then release those "stuck" emotions. Each time we are emotionally wounded, yet act as if we are not affected, we internalize those emotions, thus wounding our spirit. Those buried emotions stay buried within until we get in touch with them again and release them.

When a crisis occurs in a person's life, he may feel as though he has hit bottom, gone as far as he can go. He now truly wants to put himself in God's hands for guidance and help. This may become a turning point in a person's life. Years earlier, I had an extraordinary experience occur, which I feel caused much of my inner healing to begin. I decided to enroll in a one-night course on self-hypnosis to relieve stress. Although I did not feel I was under undue stress, I became very intrigued by the course title.

The teacher began the class by giving background information on how hypnosis works, the different levels the mind goes through to obtain the hypnotic state, and how it can benefit a person in relieving stress or removing a negative habit such as smoking. He explained the brain waves in a conscious, hypnotic, and sleeping state. Since I have always been curious how things work, I found this information very interesting. The teacher became irritated with several of the students who said, "He should get on with the hypnosis and forget the nonsense information." He became disgruntled with their attitude and immediately prepared us for our first group hypnotic session.

After the instructor induced the group into a hypnotic state, he asked the students to individually blow up a big blue balloon and then tie a white ribbon around the balloon. Next, we were instructed to tie the other end of the ribbon around our wrist. At this point, he said that the large balloon would make our arm rise up. No matter how hard I tried, my arm refused to move. Still under hypnosis, I remember feeling I was not following his instructions adequately because my arm would not go up! After he brought us out of hypnosis, I asked him why my arm wouldn't budge. He gave me a strange look, then stated that I'm the type of person who does not want to be controlled, which is why I wouldn't listen to his command and raise my arm when instructed to do so. That was a revelation!

All the years growing up, I had an extremely controlling father. At the time of the class, I was in a marriage of twenty years in which my husband controlled me. I didn't like it but was unable to stand up to my father in my earlier years, nor to stand up at that time to my husband. Yet with my subconscious in control, I was a completely different person than I appeared to be in my conscious state.

The instructor said that he would now hypnotize us to help us relax. We were all to think of a special place, real or imagined, where we would like to go to be completely comfortable and at peace. After being at this special place for a few minutes, when we came out of the hypnotic state we would all feel completely rested as though we had been asleep for ten hours. This kind of rest after only a few minutes sounded great! But for me to find a special place of comfort and peace would be difficult. I've never found a place I felt was perfect. Even though I was uncomfortable for long periods of time in the hot sun, ocean, or sand, I decided my place of peace would be at the beach, since we had taken our children there each year on vacation. This was always a time my husband and children had great fun and since their enjoyment became my enjoyment, this was where I consciously decided I would go as my special place of peace. He instructed us to breathe deeply and relax, and then put the group into a hypnotic state, this time deeper than before. When he instructed the group to go to our special place, I started to think of my peaceful place. Before I knew it, I was whisked into a dark, slightly winding tunnel and at the end was a bright glow. It all happened in a flash! There I was bathed in the most brilliant light I had ever seen. About ten feet in front and slightly above me stood Jesus, arms slightly raised with two angels in the background, one on either side. His head down to his waist was clearly visible yet faded into nothingness as I looked toward his feet. He was looking downward with a serenity I have never seen. I felt so completely enveloped as though a soft, warm, gentle blanket was slowly being placed over me completely enveloping me with an incredible, unconditional love and sense of comfort. I felt as though I had become one with the universe. Going through the tunnel, being with Jesus and so deeply emerged in his love happened within a split second.

Suddenly a realization came over me that I wasn't supposed to be there! My body jolted and I was fully awake! Everyone else was still hypnotized. It was a feeling of love that so overwhelmed me, I couldn't contain myself; my body began heaving and I began crying violently. I ran out of the room sobbing, afraid I would disturb others, still unable to control myself. After three or four minutes, I was finally able to gain control of my tears. Then within a few minutes, I began crying uncontrollably again. This went on for at least one-half hour. When I finally regained my composure, I returned to the classroom.

Shortly after my return, the class was dismissed. The instructor was concerned about my well-being and asked me to stay longer. As I began to tell him of my experience that same feeling of unconditional love came over me and I began crying again. Through my tears, I was finally able to tell him what had happened, and that I was overwhelmed with happiness. He said sometimes Jesus allows a person to be with him for a brief period of time, letting the person feel his love and know he is with them, but they cannot stay. Feeling this indescribable love caused a transformation within, which put me on the pathway to spiritual and emotional healing.

Over the past few years, several of my clients have been guided by their subconscious to go back to the time Jesus Christ walked the earth. Many of those who were friends or knew of him during that time had difficulty understanding why God would allow such pain to be bestowed upon His only Son. I have included some of these among the following sessions.

LOUISE

Louise was a quiet woman in her late forties. She had a comfortable life and good job, but said that throughout her life she had an underlying feeling of sadness and abandonment. She kept saying, "Something wants to come out." After putting Louise in a deep hypnotic state, I took her back to the cause of her sadness and feelings of abandonment.

D: Look around. Describe what you see.

L: (Softly speaks.) Carefully turning around, I feel like I am not on the Earth – some spirit place.

D: Allow yourself to be there; let the information come forward. Look up at yourself and tell me what you see. Look up from your feet.

L: White robe, white dress.

D: Feel your essence; are you male or female?

L: Female. I have blonde hair.

D: Approximately how old are you?

L: Twenty-five or twenty-eight.

D: And what are you called; what is your name?

L: Sarah Rose.

D: Look around and describe what you see.

L: It's busy, lots of people coming and going.

D What is the area called?

L: Heaven? I don't know, some spirit place.

D: And what is the time frame?

L: There is no time.

D: Look around. Is there anyone near you?

L: There is a man. He knows me but I don't know him.

D: What is he called?

L: Thomas.

D: Ask him, what does he represent to you?

L: Teaching, a guide.

D: What is he a guide for?

L: My journey.

D: Ask Thomas why he has brought you forth to him now.

L: Go – come to the earth, but I don't want to go, but I have to go.

D: Why do you not want to go?

L: I'm afraid.

D: What makes you afraid?

L: I know it is going to be hard.

D: Is there any more information?

L: God said I had to go, but I don't want to go.

D: Why did God say you have to go? What is the learning in it?

L: My soul. He wants me to come higher; he wants me to be closer; some things to get out of the way.

D: What are those things that you need to get out of the way?

L: I have to believe it is possible; it's possible.

D: And what do you have to believe is possible?

L: That He really loves me, really loves me.

D: Are you learning that in your current lifetime?

L: Yes, yes.

D: Tell me what is going on.

L: I am not finished.

D: This place you called heaven, a spirit place. Is this prior to your current lifetime or another time?

L: This time, oh. (Long pause.)

D: Where are you? Describe what is going on.

L: It is very bright, dry, hot climate, very sunny. It's a caravan. I am traveling with a caravan, going someplace.

D: Where are you going?

L: To get food. There is no food. We are going to get some food.

D: Are you still in this place called heaven, a spirit place?

L: No, no.

D: Go to a significant event. Tell me what is going on.

L: (Pause.) Some kind of trial. There's a lot of people around, yelling, shouting.

D: Go up to the trial. Go closer, go closer. Tell me what is going on. What is this trial about? Allow it to come forward; you can analyze it later. (Louise begins fidgeting, heavy breathing.) If you need to view it as a movie, allow yourself to do so. (Louise begins sniffing.) If you need to go through it, then allow yourself to do so. It is your choice. (She gasps and starts to cry as I'm speaking.)

L: (Crying and yelling.) They are hurting my friend!

D: Why are they hurting your friend?

L: (Sobbing.) They said they, they are hurting him because he tried to tell them the truth.

D: Who is your friend?

L: (Sobbing.) His name is Jesus.

D: Allow the pain to come forward. Allow yourself to release the pain; you no longer need to hold onto the pain, you have the memories. Keep releasing the pain from your body. (Her breathing is heavy as she is releasing.) Keep releasing it. And now continue.

L: (In a loud voice.) Why is this happening to him? Why are you letting this happen to him?

D: What is the response?

L: (Begins calming down.) Just a bigger picture.

D: Are you allowed to see the bigger picture?

L: Yes.

D: Then allow it to come forward.

L: It is allowing peace to come to the world. It is about healing coming into the world, to let love come into the world. It's an act of love.

D: Then ask your Higher Self and subconscious, are you accepting of all these reasons?

L: I understand, but I am still mad at the pain he was caused.

D: Where are you holding onto that anger in your body, in your physical body?

L: Chest.

D: Then go into your chest. Go into the chest area and gather up all the anger. Look deeply into that anger and allow it to come forward. What is coming forward with that anger?

L: If God could do this to him, he could do it to me.

D: Keep bringing forth the information.

L: I don't like this kind of love. I don't want to suffer like that.

D: Digging deep into the anger, is it combined with the feeling of abandonment?

L: Yes.

D: Then allow it to come forward. What is coming forward from the abandonment?

L: He left me in pain, left me in pain. He left me to experience pain.

D: Allow yourself to gather up all the abandonment feelings and the anger that is left over, the remnants in your chest area, and imagine gathering them up in your hands. Imagine your hands scooping deep within your body, gathering it all up and gently giving it back. Give it back. You no longer need to hold onto it. You now understand the reasoning. Are you giving it back? (Louise shakes head slightly up and down with hands moving as though scooping from body and pushing into the air.) Continue to give it back until it is all gone. Let me know when you are finished.

L: It is done.

(Cleansed area with healing water; filled it with pink representing love.)

D: What were the lessons that you learned from that lifetime?

L: Things sometimes are different than they look like. It was only my perception that God didn't love me. God loves me. He didn't leave me. He didn't leave me.

D: And how does that make you feel?

L: Peaceful.

D: Then allow that peaceful feeling to grow with you, that feeling of being at peace. Imagine now looking up at the light, and allow yourself to go toward the light. Feel your physical body, your spirit going through the light. And as you do, imagine yourself being cleansed from any negativity from that lifetime. Take with you only the positive and all the learning's from that lifetime. And now, allow yourself to be through the light on the other side. (Louise takes a deep breath.) Allow Thomas to come forward again to be here with you. (Pause.) Is he here with you?

L: Yes.

D: And what would you like to say to Thomas now?

L: You were right. Thank you. (Weeping softly, sniffing.)

D: If you would like to hug him or hold him, allow yourself to do so. Feel his energies always with you, beside you, guiding you. You now know in your current lifetime, even though you may not be aware of the big picture, God is always with you. Thomas is always with you. You are being guided along your path. All the feelings of abandonment are gone. Is there anything else that Thomas would like you to know before you leave?

L: He asked me to trust him and to let him help me.

D: Do you accept this?

L: Yes, oh yes!

End of session.

Louise no longer felt alone and helpless without a man in her life. She said it was as though a heavy weight had been lifted. She felt lighter and in control of herself, something that had escaped her for many years. In addition, Louise had many times questioned her confused feelings about God and religion not understanding why, as she stated, "I was always so mad at God, but didn't know why."

Ernest Pecci, M.D. states: "Regression therapy is helpful because it loosens the rigidity of the intellect and opens the door to a new experience of reality. In it one experiences a body that has been conditioned by a somewhat different personality configuration, and one becomes able to see the arbitrary nature of the current personality." This heightened awareness then makes possible a review of the current life from a more objective perspective. As a problem or symptom is experienced, eliminating the symptom might not be so important as understanding what we need to know to bring us to that place of peace and harmony with the inner self that will enable us to live more fully.

Sonja

Sonja complained of a deep, inner loneliness. She would be in a crowd, yet still felt all alone. At birthday parties where she was the center of attention with all her friends around, she felt a void within down to her depths almost as though it were, as she said, "a spiritual sacrifice."

Once Sonja was in a deep hypnotic state, we began:

D: Imagine going back in time to the cause of a deep inner loneliness, a feeling of spiritual sacrifice, and allow yourself to be there, another time, another place. Allow it to come into focus. Imagine looking down at your feet and tell me what you see.

S: I have brown sandals on, and so does Jesus.

D: What are you called?

S: Mary.

D: How are you feeling with Jesus?

S: It was a setup, for he is about to die, and I know it is going to happen. He knows what's going to happen. It is part of the way, it is part of the way he uses to teach. Even though we know it will have an impact on the minds of men, there is a heavy sadness.

D: Then I ask your subconscious and your Higher Self, is it time to remove this heavy sadness?

S: Yes.

D: Where are you holding onto this heavy sadness?

S: (Pause.) My jaw and my face, my cheeks, my tears won't stop flowing.

D: Allow yourself to completely encircle the entire area of your jaw, your cheeks, your face, your tears. Completely encircle them. If you would give this heavy sadness a color, what color would it be?

S: Gray.

D: Allow this gray to fill the entire area, completely enveloping the sadness. Begin blowing it out your mouth, (she blows it out her mouth) going into Mother Earth. Continue removing it. (Again takes a deep breath, blowing.) See the gray diminishing, removing all the sadness. (Continues to take deep breaths and blowing.) Has it all been removed?

S: Yes.

(I now have her cleanse herself internally with healing water, filling the area with peachy orange and joy as she requested.)

D: Before you leave, is there anything you would like to say to Jesus?

S: (Long pause.) I would like to thank him for the lessons. They are the depth of conviction of his soul, of what he had to do for the many and not for himself, to use his life for them.

D: Is there anything he would like to say to you before he leaves?

S: I need to understand, as I often knew, it was his job and not mine – my solar plexus, so alone.

D: Go into the solar plexus, all the way to the cause of feeling alone.

S: I'm afraid. He's gone.

D: Allow (Sonja cuts me off as I'm speaking.)

S: He's gone. I feel lonely.

D: Go into the solar plexus. Go all the way to the cause of feeling alone, the lonely feeling of him being gone. Begin pushing it out.

S: (Moans and groans.)

D: Tell me what is going on.

S: It won't leave this area. I think I was wounded.

D: Go into the cause of feeling like you were wounded.

S: A knife – sword.

D: Allow it to come into focus. Tell me what happened.

S: I got in the way.

D: You got in the way of what?
S: I tried to stop it.
D: What did you try to stop?
S: A stab.
D: And who stabbed you with a sword?
S: A soldier.
D: Was your death caused by the stab wound?
S: Yes.
D: Give it back to him. It is time to remove it. Has it been removed? Tell me what is going on.
S: It moves.
D: Find it. Keep removing it. Allow the pain to come out of the opening where the sword went in. Allow it to flow freely, out that wounded area, onto the floor, removing that pain. As it flows out, what would you like to tell that soldier?
S: You don't understand what you're doing! You have to know the cause. He is not your enemy.
D: Keep allowing it to drain out. You no longer need to hold onto the pain.
S: Okay.
D: Allow the golden-white light representing purity to completely fill the area where you were wounded because of your love for Jesus. Feel the energies growing stronger and stronger and stronger within you, with a knowing that Jesus is always with you. He may have died a physical death, but he has always been with you spiritually. Knowing this, you no longer have to feel lonely. He has always been with you. His love for you has always been there. Allow his love to regenerate you. Allow that love to grow within you and as it does, allow your body to heal. Feel the healing taking place.
S: (Keeps coughing, clearing throat.)
D: Is there any other significant event in that lifetime that you need to go to?

S: There's the one group of women.

D: Then allow yourself to be there. What is the significance of this group of women?

S: They are all followers, too.

D: Walk around. Look at each one, feel their essence. Look into their eyes. Do you recognize any of them in your current life-time?

S: Yes.

D: Then allow yourself to bring forth the recognition.

S: There is Joanna and Heather and Judy. They're here for energy and support.

D: Why are they showing themselves at this time? Ask your subconscious.

S: I understand a collective gathering again.

D: It is also a knowing that you are no longer alone, you have never been alone; they have always been there with you. Is there any information you would like to bring forward into your current lifetime from that lifetime?

S: There will always be those who disagree, who can't know, don't want to know – the soldiers, the people who oppose, the people who can't see the truth.

D: Is there any more information to be brought forth?

S: No, I now know.

End of session.

In discussion after the session, Sonja said her name, Mary, was very common in those days. She was not Mary Magdalene, but she was a friend of Jesus. During the time of the crucifixion, she said some of the other women contained themselves, but she couldn't. She was upset by what the soldiers were doing, tried to stop them, and was killed for interfering. The soldiers were very stoic; they were there just to do a job. She said when she went into the light after her death, Jesus was waiting for her putting his hand on her wound.

Sonja had a dull ache in the area where the sword was inflicted in that lifetime, but did not mention it prior to hypnosis. The ache has since disappeared along with the deeper inner void of loneliness.

JENNIFER

Jennifer, a strikingly beautiful redhead with light blue eyes, years earlier had been diagnosed with fibromyalgia. She complained of pain and tenderness in her joints, fought bouts of depression, and at times was "just plain fatigued." She said the symptoms would "just come and go." After Jennifer was in a hypnotic state, the following session unfolded:

D: Scan your body. Where are you holding onto fibromyalgia? Go into your body and allow your subconscious to do the work.

J: Legs and feet.

D: Go into your feet. Go into your feet as you continue to go down deeper and deeper. Can you see the fibromyalgia in your feet?

J: Yes.

D: Go into it and become a part of it. Become part of it and let it take you where it will.

J: It doesn't seem to be taking me anywhere.

D: Ask your subconscious; is your conscious fighting this?

J: I don't know. Nothing is happening.

D: Ask your conscious; is it getting in the way?

J: I think it could be.

D: Why? Ask it why.

J: I don't want to go back.

D: Go back where?

J: To the time of Jesus.

D: Why?

J: I didn't like it.

D: What is the obstacle? Ask your subconscious if it is time to go back to the time of Jesus to resolve some of the problems that you have been holding onto.

J: Well, I get yes, but – (Long pause.)

D: Allow yourself to go back in time. Is part of your fibromyalgia caused by your lifetime during the time of Christ?

J: Yes.

D: Allow yourself to go back to that time. It is time to release the pain caused by that lifetime.

J: Okay.

D: Now look at yourself. Tell me what you see.

J: It seems like I'm in a prison or something, or jail.

D: What do you look like? Look at yourself and describe yourself.

J: I don't know.

D: Are you female or male?

J: I think I'm female. I don't know why I'm not getting it very clear though.

D: Don't try to analyze it. You can analyze it later. Look around. Is there anyone with you?

J: Yeah, there are some other people.

D: Is there anyone next to you?

J: There's a man.

D: Why is he there?

J: We're actually both here because we've got to fight with the lions.

D: And why do you have to go out and fight the lions?

J: We're Christians and we're supposed to. One of us has to go, and so he's going to go instead of me.

D: And why is that? Who decided that?

J: He did. He doesn't want me to die.

D: What is his relationship to you?

J: He's my lover. I don't know what this has to do with Jesus. (Long pause.)

D: You can analyze this later. Let me do the work. Continue to go down, down. What is your name?

J: Sophia.
D: How old are you Sophia?
J: Twenty-three.
D: And your lover, what is his name?
J: Claudius.
D: What are your feelings toward him?
J: I don't think I love him very much, because I let him die.
D: Go into your feelings. Go into your feelings and emotions and tell me what you are feeling.
J: I'm just feeling scared.
D: Go into feeling scared. Are there any other emotions?
J: I feel guilty because we were both supposed to go out, and he's going by himself. I don't know how they let me have a choice in the matter though.
D: And why were you sent there to fight the lions?
J: I'm a Christian. I am a Christian.
D: Do you believe you are a true Christian?
J: (Deep sigh.) No, because I'm scared and I don't want to die.
D: And how does that make your feel?
J: Terrible, but I just don't want to die.
D: Go into being a Christian and being scared and afraid of dying. Go into all those feelings.
J: I feel like a failure because I should be willing to die for Jesus. I just don't want to die. I guess I don't believe enough.
D: Do you feel like you betrayed Jesus?
J: Yes.
D: Go into that feeling of betrayal. Go deep into that feeling of betrayal. What other emotions is it bringing up?
J: (Breathing heavy.) Sorrow, failure. I know I failed.
D: Is it time to remove these feelings from your body?
J: Yes.
D: Where are you holding onto these feelings?

J: My neck and shoulders and my hands, my feet. (Takes a deep breath.) I just saw him torn up by the lions. I don't really like it very much. (Long pause.)

D: Continue. Tell me what is going on.

J: Nothing. They let me go because I renounced my faith.

D: How does that make you feel?

J: (Several deep breaths.) Horrible.

D: Go into that feeling. Do you feel they were right in forcing you to die by lions because of your faith?

J: NO! I don't think people should die like that.

D: Is it time to remove those negative feelings? They were at fault, not you.

J: Yes. I would like to get rid of them.

D: Then scan your entire body. As I point out the feelings within your body, find them. Find sorrow, the feelings of betrayal, pain, anger, guilt. Are there any other feelings? Scan your body; take your time.

J: Sad. I felt very sad.

D: Find where you are holding onto the sadness. Now ask your angels and your guides to do a cleanup on your body, removing all those negative feelings from that lifetime, a lifetime where others were at fault, not you. They were trying to rid you of your beliefs, your religion.

J: Yes.

D: Ask your guides and angels to come in and start at the top of your head and do a complete and total cleansing. Are your guides here?

J: Yes.

D: Imagine yourself being cleansed, beginning with your head, slowly and gently flowing down through your body, as you remove all the negative emotions and feelings from that lifetime, a lifetime where they were wrong, not you. Now allow the cleansing to flow into your heart, removing the sadness from your heart, your arms, flowing down your arms, (Jennifer coughs loudly several times) removing all those negative feelings you've carried for so long. Now your hands, taking extra time working on your hands. Keep removing the build-up of illness within your body caused by holding onto this. Continue down your upper back and your lower back. Continue down to your hips, allowing the cleansing to flow to all the areas of your body, cleansing and healing your body, healing your body from that lifetime. Your body is ridding itself of those negative emotions. Down, down, down to your feet. Do some extra work with your feet. When you are completely finished let me know. Take your time.

J: (Long pause.) I think I'm finished.

D: Is there anything from that lifetime that your subconscious wants to address at this time?

J: (Deep breath.) I feel like it's time to leave. I didn't like going there in the first place.

D: Then allow yourself to leave. Allow yourself to look up, going to the white light.

(Finished taking her through the white light for further cleansing and healing.)

End of session.

It has been over five years since Jennifer's session. Her fibromyalgia lessened for a while, then came back. In my summation, Jennifer is still holding onto some guilt, never completely forgiving herself for renouncing her Christianity.

CHAPTER 5

ATTACHMENT

The condition of spirit possession – that is, full or partial takeover of a living human by a discarnate being – has been recognized or at least theorized in every era and every culture. In ninety percent of societies worldwide there are records of possession-like phenomena (Foulks, 1985).

The following case is an example of how an unknown spirit attachment can affect a person's physical and mental well-being.

Erin

Erin was a soft-spoken woman in her mid-forties. "My body is breaking down," she said. Other comments were, "I feel tired all the time and I'm worried about my health. I think my pituitary gland is failing. My third eye keeps tingling. I keep putting on weight. I've put on fifty pounds in the past ten years. My headaches are getting worse. The doctors can't find anything wrong. I don't know what to do anymore."

After inducing a deep hypnotic state, we began:

D: Allow yourself to go within and find your pituitary gland. Tell me what it looks like.

E: I don't know what it's supposed to look like.

D: Just look at it, allowing the information to come forward.

E: It's very pale, and tired.

D: What is causing the pituitary gland to feel tired?

E: It has to do too much work. It's feeling like it's all by itself.

D: Go deep within the cause. Why does it feel like it's all by itself?

E: Because it's broken.

D: What is causing it to be broken?

E: I am.

D: Why are you causing it to be broken?

E: I'm too busy.

D: What are you too busy doing?

E: Everything. It's just such a big job for it.

D: Ask your subconscious. What can you do so it does not feel so overworked?

E: I need to sleep.

D: Will sleep help the pituitary gland grow stronger?

E: It will help me.

D: By helping you, how will it help the pituitary gland?

E: If I sleep, I don't worry about anything.

D: Go to the cause of your worries. What is causing all your worries?

E: (Deep sigh.) I think it's about my mother. (Erin's mother died in the 1980s.)

D: I ask your mother to come forward and be here with you. Allow her to be here with you. Is she coming forth?

E: She's just holding on.

D: What is she holding onto?

E: Me.

D: Why is she holding onto you?

E: I can't tell. She's dark.

D: Ask her why she's dark.

E: She's hiding.

D: Ask her to come forth into the light. Why is she hiding?

E: She doesn't want anybody to know she's here.

D: Why does she not want anyone to know she's here?

E: She's still angry and she's confused.

D: I ask your mother if she would allow me to talk to her.

E: She's afraid.

D: What is she afraid of?

E: You won't like her.

D: She is on the spirit side. She can see me. She knows that I will not judge her.

E: She's not there.

D: Scan your body. Has your mother attached to any part of your body?

E: (Deep breath.) In my mid-section.

D: Go into your mid-section and ask your mother to come forth.

E: She's here now.

D: Why is she attached to your mid-section?

E: She won't let go of this life.
D: Why won't she let go of this life?
E: She wasn't finished.
D: What was left unfinished?
E: She never got to be happy.
D: Ask her if I can help her in any way to go to the other side where she will be happy.
E: She's listening.
D: I am here, and if she will allow herself to look up toward the Light, I will help guide her to the Light.
E: She's changing colors.
D: Imagine now, gently leaving this physical form, going up toward the Light, and I will help guide you to the Light.
E: She's unfolding, but she's still holding onto me.
D: I ask that she keep looking up toward the Light. The Light will help cleanse her from the negativity. It will help brighten her; it will help lighten her load. Allow her to continue toward the Light. If she wishes to go in slow increments, that is fine, a portion at a time. If this is easier for her, allow her to do so.
E: (Begins fidgeting.) I want her to go.
D: Is there anything she would like to tell you, or discuss with you before she goes to the Light that will help release her?
E: She doesn't have a lot of good things to say.
D: Is there anything you would like to tell her that will help release her?
E: I want her to go. I want her to go.
D: After she goes to the Light, she will be at peace on the other side, and she can still come back to you from the other side.
E: (Pause.) I told her she can go.
D: I ask her now if she is ready to go to the Light. If she would like, allow my energies to go forth to help carry her to the Light.
E: She's still holding.

D: I ask that she release herself from you. Allow your spirituality to help her go to the Light.

E: (Moves hands as though she's trying to pull something off body.) She's only holding me in one place. It's like she's made of rubber.

D: It is time to go to the Light. It is okay. She can do much healing on the other side where she will have great help and guidance. (Pause.) I now ask her guide to come forth to help guide her to the other side.

E: Yes, but she's scared of him. Are you sure that's where he's from?

D: Allow her guide to come forth. Ask him if he is her guide.

E: (Gasps.) He said she belongs to him!

D: I ask in the name of Jesus Christ, who are you?! Are you from the Light?!

E: No!

D: Where are you from?

E: He's from nowhere.

D: Ask her guide from the Christ energy to come forth to help her.

E: Oh my goodness! That's why she was afraid to leave. Okay. (Loud voice.) He's trying to get to her!

D: The Light is stronger than darkness!

E: (Loud groan.) I have to move this other fella.

D: Allow the energy from the Christ Light to grow stronger and stronger, cutting away and dimming the blackness, as though you were going into a room that is dark and turning on the light switch, and now the room is bright. Light is stronger than darkness!

E: (Sigh). He gets it now.

D: Allow the Christ energy to now come forth.

E: He took her by the arm.

D: Allow the Christ energy to surround her so that she knows she is safe and being guided.

E: She's still crying. She's afraid. It's okay; it's okay.

D: She is now being guided by the Christ energy.

E: (Pause.) She'll be all right. She's now going forward. (Whispering.) She's so sad. I feel sorry for her.

D: She has made her own choices in her lifetime.

E: (Deep sigh, long pause.)

D: It is time to release all negative thoughts and feelings. (Deep sighs coming from Erin). You no longer need to hold on to any negative energies. Feel them being released from you.

E: (Sobbing.) She had such a tragic life.

D: She helped to make you who you are. It is time to continue to release all negative energies caused by her.

E: Is there any way to keep her from coming back?

D: She has crossed over into the Light.

E: She's done it before, but she comes back.

D: Imagine a beautiful golden glow from above, from the spirit side, the Christ energy. Allow this golden glow to come down over you, passing through you, protecting you. This is a protective shield that she cannot penetrate. She is being taken care of on the spirit side. She can no longer come back and attach to you. It is now time for you to continue forward in your destiny. This golden glow is completely impenetrable; it is sealing you in the Light. Know from within that it is sealed tightly. Your guides are here with you to help. (Pause.) You may now walk freely, having released all negative energies caused by your mother. Feel your body becoming lighter. (Pause.) You have learned from her, positive and negative, and now you no longer need her energies. Allow your physical form to glow and be sealed in the Light. She can no longer reattach to you or harm you in any way. Allow it to be a known from within.

E: Okay. (Deep sigh.)

D: Tell me what is going on.

E: I have my family around me, and I have my angels. They told me I'm like a sponge. I take whatever is hurting her. I wanted to help her, and she just attached to me. But I have to stop doing that. People have to help themselves (sigh).

D: It has been twenty-five years since your mother has passed away. You have helped her enough. You have now released her so that she may do her own work.

E: Her mother's going to be with her for a while. She'll be okay now. She's got her mom.

D: Know that if you would even think of bringing her back, it would not help her. It would set her back.

E: I don't want to – I want her to go on her own. She's gone now.

D: Does your physical form feel lighter?

E: Oh, yes.

D: Scan your physical form. Have you released all the negative energies from her?

E: Yeah!

(Erin was instructed to go out into the universe, among the beauty of the stars, to rest for a moment. Then we continued.)

D: Bring all your attention to your third eye.

E: It hurts.

D: Go to the cause of the hurting.

E: I don't know. There's something wrong. I'm afraid, but there's a growth on there.

D: Go to the cause of thinking there is a growth on your third eye. Is there a growth on your third eye?

E: Yes. The system's failing.

D: What is causing your system to fail?

E: Age. It's faster than normal.

D: I ask your guide to come forth to be here with you.

E: I see a very bright light over the pain. He's more than a guide.

D: Tell me in detail, what information is coming forth?

E: The Master Teacher is here. (Pause.) There are so many things I have to experience here. I'm experiencing them in my spiritual growth, but I also have to do it in this body. The discomfort's just a test. By slowly breaking down the body and changing, you learn more about who you really are. It's been difficult. It's difficult to love yourself, so when you're without your body it's much easier, so the body is breaking down quickly. It's not necessarily a bad thing, though. And there's no such thing as a wasted life, no matter how little you think you may have accomplished. All lives take steps forward in great strides, even the most humble person. An awakened body isn't necessarily a sign of an awakened spirit, no matter what people want to tell you. It doesn't mean that you're spiritually weak; it only means that your physical body is weak. (Takes a deep breath.) I agreed to this! It's just that I'd forgotten that it would come quickly. It's all right. I'm surrounded with people who love me, not just in the physical, and he's with me all the time. He says it's a good thing that my mother's gone. It was good to help her. She was just very, very frightened, but she'll be protected. He says I shouldn't be pushing my luck.

D: What does he mean by pushing your luck?

E: I keep asking for things. (Giggles.) He's just messing with me.

D: Does he have any information and more guidance in the work you do?

E: Yes.

D: Can that be brought forth at this time?

E: He says I know. He's provided me the information I need to do for other people.

D: Are they people you already know or will they come forth?

E: They'll come to me. One is someone I know already, but he's not going to tell me who it is. It's part of my healing work, and he's going to provide me with more opportunities for more outlets. I'm going to be working with more hospice work, but I knew that. He's moving away.

D: Thank him for sharing and bringing forth this information.

E: He knows. He loves me. I always call him Father when we talk. (Sigh.) He's taking some of the pain with him. He's leaving some, just a little as a reminder.

D: Is there any more information for you at this time?

E: No.

(I instructed Erin to put a golden healing, protective light around her, and then asked her to go to her peaceful place to rest and reenergize.)

End of session.

The discussion after the session was very interesting and I felt it added to the hypnosis, so I have included some of it.

E: (In reference to her mother.) I could see her, almost in a fetal position, completely surrounding my body, like she was made of rubber on my body. I feel lighter already. She was just so afraid, and she didn't want to leave. It was very difficult. I was trying to pull her off my body and have the guides pull her off, but her fingers would reach out and hang on tighter. She was like one of those dolls you stretch. The person waiting for her I think scared her. He was a pretty scary-looking shape. I couldn't see the face, but it was a big, dark void waiting for her. I had the feeling that that may have been of her own creation. It just kept getting bigger and bigger the more I would try to pull her off me, so she wouldn't let go. I was really glad when you starting talking her through because I could feel it helped her to go. I do feel lighter. She was just such a tragic figure. Her mother, my grandmother, was there for her and with her, and she loved her mother. She could comfort her.

My mother was a big woman. I even started looking like my mother. I never looked like my mother before! It just hit me! She may have been attached because she thought I would take her from this lifetime. I'm thinking she knew I helped her before. We know these things on another level; that's why she attached to me instead of my sister or brother because she knew I would help her. That's why when she found out how sick she was and said she's going to die, I told her I would take care of her and then it didn't happen. I don't feel bad about that now. That's good. It was emotional, but as she was pulling away, I could feel all that she was feeling. I was picturing myself like a rag, wringing myself out. It was very intense, but it was good. She was a horrible woman in this life. Not a nice person. I came in knowing there were certain things I would have to handle. Oddly, I don't feel afraid.

(In reference to her third eye.) It was amazing to feel that in my head. I get such headaches. I was happy to hear it because it bothered me that my body was breaking down. I needed to hear that. Because of all the things I was studying, I thought my body should be in much better shape, and now I understand I am spiritually growing.

D: You need to trust your inner self. Some people mean well, but it's not coming forth accurately.

E: I keep thinking it's because I'm not spiritual enough, or focused enough; but now I know that our relationship with our Creator is very personal; each one is different.

In the follow-up a week later, Erin said she weighed herself the evening after the hypnosis and had dropped two pounds. The next morning, she dropped another two pounds! She has not had another headache and her energy is increasing.

"Earthbound spirits, the surviving consciousness of deceased humans, are the most prevalent possessing, obsessing or attaching entities to be found," according to Dr. William Baldwin in his book, *Spirit Releasement Therapy.* He continues:

> The disembodied consciousness seems to attach itself and merge fully or partially with the subconscious mind of a living person, exerting some degree of influence on thought processes, emotions, behavior and the physical body. The entity becomes a parasite in the mind of the host. The host is usually unaware of the presence of attached spirits. The thoughts, desires and behaviors of an attached entity are experienced as the person's own thoughts, desires and behaviors. Many spirits remain in the earth plane due to a lack of awareness of their passing. An attachment can be benevolent in nature, totally self-serving, malevolent in intention, or completely neutral. A spirit can be bound to the earth plane by the emotions and feelings connected with a sudden traumatic death. Anger, fear, jealousy, resentment, guilt, remorse, even strong ties of love can interfere with the normal transition.

In summation, many of the physical changes occurring in Erin were attributable to the attachment of her mother. Because of the "horrible" things her mother did while alive (as relayed by Erin in discussion after the hypnosis, but not included here) her mother resisted going to the Light after dying because of her fear of what she would face in the afterlife.

CHAPTER 6

EXTRATERRESTRIALS

"We are all one!" states Ruth Montgomery, once a top White House correspondent, then the author of numerous thought-provoking books channeled by her guides on paranormal and psychic topics. In *Aliens Among Us*, she continues:

> My Guides repeatedly stress that our space brothers and sisters share with us a mutual Creator, and that far from being a unique form of life in an otherwise uninhabited cosmos, we humans are comparatively backward souls who came to Schoolhouse Earth to learn much needed lessons.
>
> The more enlightened ones among us, according to the Guides, have had numerous lives on other planets as well as earth, and have returned here to rescue us from our limited thought patterns before it is too late. Some of our "unearthly" visitors, they say, have emerged from spaceships to test our environment, take samplings of our flora and fauna to reseed in other galaxies, and conduct harmless experiments with human beings, manifesting themselves and their spacecraft here by reassembling the pattern of the atoms. But a significantly larger group of spacelings, the Guides insist, volunteered to be born into earthly bodies. In other words, they are like us....

In Human Form

Sanni

In March 2003, I received a letter from a college professor, Dr. Henry, at the Eastern New Mexico University, Roswell campus. We met several months earlier in New Mexico at Sharon's home, a dear friend and mutual acquaintance. He had been interested in UFOs and anything connected with the subject for many years. Because of his interest, he was introduced to Sanni (her pseudo name), a woman in her mid-forties, who believes she is the reincarnated commander of a space ship that crashed near Roswell in 1947. He invited me to New Mexico to meet Sanni and stated, "You could hypnotize Sanni so she can tell us her story and the history of the activities of the Star People on earth with great clarity and detail."

I was intrigued, to say the least. Up to that time, I had no known dealings with extraterrestrials. He said, "Sanni must be handled very carefully because she is frightened of psychiatrists and counselors. She is racked with pain and anguish over the ship's crash and the death of her shipmates." He states he has, "Verified she could fluently write the symbolic universal language. This language is so complex that it has baffled a colleague of mine here at the University who is an expert in languages and cryptography. We compared her writing to that found in a crashed space ship and it is identical!"

Dr. Henry believed a casual, home setting would be best so as not to frighten Sanni. A date was set up three weeks in the future at Sharon's home in New Mexico. I put aside the entire weekend for my trip. As I arrived at her home, Sharon greeted me with a warm welcome. Several hours later we received a call from Dr. Henry, who had just arrived at a local hotel with Sanni. He wanted to share some of Sanni's background before we met her. "There seems to be nothing that I can do to keep her from feeling sorry for herself," he said, "but when she begins to talk about the Star people and their activities in space, her knowledge is very extensive and appears to be coming from a very advanced spirit."

Sharon and I decided to meet Sanni for a short time that evening so she could become comfortable with new people in her life. Dr. Henry suggested she not be told about my field of work that evening so she would not be frightened further.

When Sanni walked through the door, I was greeted with a physically frail, hunched-over woman appearing older than her years. Her shoulder-length hair was completely white, her skin was the color of an albino, and she had large, piercing, dark-brown eyes. She seemed apprehensive, hiding behind Dr. Henry as a young child who was meeting new playmates for the first time. Slowly she came forward, and as I reached out my hand touching hers, Sanni gave me a big hug and began crying. She appeared emotionally strained and tired from her long trip. She was introduced to Sharon, and began hugging and crying all over again. We sat for more than an hour, Sanni crying and holding both Sharon and me. She told me she could immediately feel people's energy, and constantly said, "She loved to feel our energy because of the love in it." As they left for the evening, Dr. Henry handed me a copy of *The Star Beacon* dated April, 1999, which contained an article written about Sanni called "Stranded on Earth."

As I read the four-page article, I couldn't help question what I was reading, but I kept an open mind. The article states, "She is a star person living among us. Her mother was selected to have her; alien DNA genetic material would be implanted into her and she would have a hybrid being. Sanni was the first batch of hybrids

– Alpha beings – those who could live on this planet, but with some difficulty." The article continued with Sanni's words:

I am almost paranoid of what people will think. They may feel I am a mental-ward case. I am not. I am a VISITOR. I do not want to be here. It was extreme karmic punishment. I was not supposed to lead an expedition to this solar system of Terra. I disobeyed the Council of Galactic Light (or Grays' version of Interplanetary United Worlds or Nations). (There was to be) no interference in a primitive or warlike planet. No trade, no relations or landings were to be made upon a backward species planet. I came here because I was a scientist, and I caused the accident that ended my 'life' and the lives of five members of my crew. I didn't pay attention to the instruments, and this created loss of shields and defenses around our vehicle. An electrical storm on your Terra knocked out the ship's force fields. We crashed in the desert with liquid pouring from the skies of Terra. I only survived about a month in your Terran time.

I remember being thrown out of our vehicle and a big explosion ripped a hole. This caused scattering of machinery and crew out onto Terra's desert. People were crying and in pain. I was badly hurt, and at that time I realized I'd broken Prime Directive One rules, as stated via the Council in our own home world. I was taken to the "hospital" or facility. I didn't understand English, as we didn't have a universal language translator device or ULTD on our uniforms. I was badly burned on the left side, my leg, arm, and head. I was in bad pain. Earth creatures gave me nothing to alleviate it. Earth creatures were bigger than me. They interrogated me by using nine specialists who knew telepathy. They asked questions, such as why we came here, were we hostile, did we have war, and did we have religion? I was a guinea pig to Earth creatures. They poked, prodded, stuck things (tubes) into me, touched me, and also abused me when they tried to determine if I was a male or female entity (I was a female). I cannot put into English how much I hurt and how I regretted what I did.

Dr. Henry and Sanni arrived late the following morning accompanied by Dr. Henry's fiancée, Erica. Sanni immediately hugged Sharon, then hugged me and sat down beside me, holding my hand. At one point, she pulled up her pant leg and said, "Look, Dr. D., my skin is white and I have no hair on my arms or legs!" She then motioned for me to touch her skin. It felt very slick, like smooth, shiny silk. Although she physically appeared elderly, emotionally she acted like a young child, and was excited when Dr. Henry brought out blank paper and markers. As we casually talked, I asked Sanni if she would write something for me in her language. She was quite agreeable, and even drew pictures of her ship. Her writing consisted of symbols and hieroglyphics. As she continued drawing the inner workings of her ship, she began telling me about "her story," the fatal crash.

Now it was time I explained my profession to her. As I did, I asked if she would like me to hypnotize her to help release some of her emotional pain from the crash in 1947. "Oh, could you?" She exclaimed. "But I don't want to forget what happened. I miss them so much. But I don't want this pain anymore," she said as she held my hand, not wanting to let go. As we sat, I began talking to her, putting her into a restful hypnotic state, which she went into easily.

The following is what came forth under hypnosis:

D: Tell me where you are. What is going on?

S: (Unfamiliar language spoken that I did not understand. In order to condense, I will refer to it as UL. Sanni later told me it was her people's language.) Capacity 6 to 12 passengers. (UL) Generators complete. Standby. Operational reactive matter, anti-matter reactive pulsed? (I couldn't understand this word.) Fusion, titanium, (UL) platinum, (UL) platinum, titanium, aluminum. (UL)

Interface with computer modulator mentally. (UL) Mothership released into atmosphere, high atmosphere, (UL) intermediate phase, (UL), equipped with right pods in case of emergency; left pods contain capsule. Each crewmember get into pod and eject as pilot ejects from ship is part of plan B. The other wing of the first pod, ship carried on large mothership, see number eight in succession. This is a small-class anti-vessel originating in (unfamiliar word) but also used as (unfamiliar word) and the Pleiadians and other species. (UL) Research study of atom. Nuclear testing what brought us here. Man plays with atom as though it was toy. Man, earthling not understand that atom can end the life on planet as you know it. (UL) Use of atom must end soon or destruction of your solar system and the air in it will be complete. Many many many more ships shall come. Stand by, stand by to evacuate if possible all those who are seeded, all those that are of the hardwoods and the star seeds and the abductees will be evacuated off world, and then final war will commence, which your species call Armageddon. It will commence, and then your planet will be nothing but barren and lifeless. We will come back and we will terra form and recreate the solar system and make it a paradise as it was originally supposed to be by Yahweh. XXBAOTTG. Ships went down (voice becoming wobbly) due to a breakup in connection with the mind interface of the computer force field control device. When ships went down, lightening, lightening was attracted to the alon? alon? (not sure of word) charged hole which caused a mass explosion in XBAATTSU58096, which was the large carrier that had 12 passengers. (Voice becoming more anxious.) It is out of control (voice wavering) to small ship. (Beginning to sob, indistinguishable numbers being yelled, crying hard.) Ships went down! Ships went down! (UL being yelled.) HELP! HELP! (UL frantically yelled.) Mothership, mothership, no contact! (UL) (Cries uncontrollably, yelling and crying in UL.) Tayaha! Tayaha!

D: Keep it coming out. It's almost gone. Keep it coming out.

S: (Still crying uncontrollably.) I'M SORRY! I'M SORRY! Tayaha, come, I'm scared! (UL) (Still crying.) I looked up. I see through the? (UL) Save me! (UL) Oh the pain! It hurts! My side hurts, I was burned! I've been severely burned! My head hurts! I hear my people crying! (Pause.) But now it's silent, I don't hear any more crying, no more. Khinyeo, what happened, where am I, Khinyeo? (Sobbing in UL.) We crashed! And burned! I see smoke! It's smoke on the ship!!! She's burning! (Hysterically crying.) She's broken in several pieces!

(At this point, I would like to add what was occurring to me, something I have never experienced before or since. As Sanni was holding my arm and hand and releasing her pain, I began feeling her emotional trauma. She was passing her pain through me as it was being released from her. I was trying to keep my composure, yet I was sobbing, my nose was running, but I couldn't reach for a tissue. Each time I would try to release my hands from hers, she would grab me again and hold on. I was feeling the horrible emotional pain she had been enduring for many years.)

Continuing with the hypnosis:

D: Let it leave your body. Let the pain leave your body.

S: (Still loudly sobbing.) I didn't mean to crash it! I didn't mean to kill my people!

D: See the council in front of you. Ask their forgiveness.

S: (Speaking at length in UL.)

D: What are they saying to you?

S: (UL) The Supreme Matriculate? Council of the Federated Worlds of Love and Light and Universal Peace and Harmony. (Begins speaking loudly, almost yelling.) We forgive you for causing the crash (indistinguishable words) of 1947 of July of 3.

D: They forgive you. They forgive you. Feel that within you. Allow that to keep going through your body.

S: (Breathing becomes quieter, voice calming down.) But I caused it because earth was like a jewel with blue and green, like a jewel in the darkness of space, and I was attracted because of the diversity of the animals and plant life, for we did not have that on our land.

D: You were attracted to it, but you did not crash on purpose.

S: (Completely calm now.) The earth people were taking these bombs and detonating them on the white sands and out in the Pacific Ocean. I was here to wake up the people.

D: The crash is over. You did not do the crash on purpose. Scan your body from the top of your head to the bottom of your feet. Are you still holding onto pain from the crash?

S: It's guilt.

D: Where are you holding onto the guilt?

S: I disobeyed orders.

D: Where are you holding onto it? Is it in your head? (Yes) In your heart? (Yes) Your stomach? (Yes) Your legs? (Yes) Imagine a beautiful golden light completely surrounding your body, feel the golden light.

S: (Begins sobbing again.)

D: The golden light begins drawing out the guilt from your body from the crash. Can you feel the golden light drawing out the guilt?

S: (Sobbing.) Yes!

D: See it going into Mother Earth and being grounded into Mother Earth. Are you doing it?

S: Yes! I see my dad, Khinyeo, standing beside me. He's looking at me. He's here to help you. He's guiding you to help me. He has his hand pointed up to the stars and I see white energy coming out of them and going into his body and going down his arm and going through me.

D: He's taking the pain and guilt out of your body. Is it gone yet?

S: Almost.

D: Tell me when it's all gone.

S: (UL) It is gone.

D: Imagine cool, clear water. Do you like water?

S: I need water!

D: See yourself walking over to a cool, clear lake. See yourself walking into the water, completely immersing yourself in the cool, clear water, cleansing yourself completely.

S: Ooooohhhh.

D: What would you like to fill your body with now?

S: Khinyeo's love.

D: What color does Khinyeo's love represent to you?

S: Blue. I see a ship coming down over me.

(At this point, Sanni had been cleared of the emotional pain she had suffered throughout her lifetime, taking responsibility as commander of her fallen ship. Sanni now seemed to be a clear channel for more information to come through, of which I felt some should be included here:)

D: Why is the ship coming down over you?

S: She says she was sent by my people to help unify me and to protect me.

D: Allow the rays from the ship to enclose and protect you. Feel it deep within.

S: She is saying you will never, never be cut off from your people again. She is also saying that I am part of a group to planet Earth from the people of the Reticuli. That I was sent as a bridge between two solar systems and two galaxies to instill peace within the people of earth so that there is no war or hatred no more. She's saying that I am only one of the first to be sent to the earth to help the earth people to evolve. And she is saying that time on earth is getting short for the earth people and there must be many of us here to awaken and spread the light to end this oncoming catastrophe. She says there is a mothership near Jupiter but she is cloaked; she is on standby to evacuate all people if possible. She is also saying that there is a new star near Jupiter that has only been there a few of your months. It is not only a star; it is an artificial planet. It appears as a planet, but is really a ship disguised to look like a planet and it is called Niberu, the Ancient One. It will pass your earth and its nuclear reactors could ignite once it gets near your earth. That means it will change the orbit of your earth and that could bring disaster.

D: Why will that come about?

S: Because people, the people on Niberu have long been extinct and they lived inside of that ship, and all generations have died off. Now it goes in a certain orbit and it returns every couple of thousands of years to the earth's solar system.

D: Why is it here now?

S: Because changes are occurring on earth that must change, changes in your climate, changes in your society. The earth is on the brink of major changes. Major changes in your nations, major changes in everything because earth must evolve. If earth does not evolve, it will go backward and become worse. Earth is crying out for help. Earth is a living creature. The water is her blood, the land is her body, and earthlings have desecrated Mother Earth. They have turned her body, they have polluted her, and now she is making herself known, and she is telling the earth people that she will not take no more of this. This is why the weather has changed. This is why you see more seismic activity. Everything on earth has energy and has a soul and has light. Everything from the tiniest rock to the biggest tree; everything has a memory of who it was and who it will be. Everything remembers its pain and sorrow. You must all work together to heal Mother Earth, heal her resources, take away the sadness that hurts her soul. People must live together as one with love and light, united, and have unconditional love for all people, all people. When you have

> done this, then the mystery of our visiting your earth will be no longer. There will be no more secrecy about our ships being here among you. This is what we want for your earth; we want you to evolve and to be as us. We do not want your species to become extinct due to carelessness and war and greed, for that is not why we created your species. We created your species to evolve and to be like the rest of us, to have intergalactic space flight and to explore and to see the wonders that we have seen. We will be watching over your earth and we will be monitoring your activities.

End of hypnosis.

I have had the opportunity of meeting with Sanni several times since. A few months later, she was encouraged by Dr. Henry to go to a healing retreat in the hills of McKnight Canyon in New Mexico. This was a small retreat being held at a remote site within the canyon where healers of varied modalities come together to help those in need. Sanni came up to me, gave me a big hug, and said, "Dr. D, you helped me so much. I don't feel bad no more because of the ship crashing. Could you get rid of my hurt from when I was young?" During the course of the week's retreat, Sanni and I spent much time together, along with a session to remove her childhood emotional scars.

In conclusion, it is not for me to decide if Sanni is a Star Seed Child and former commander of a space ship that crashed in Roswell, New Mexico in 1947. What is important is the emotional state Sanni was in when I first met her and the changes that occurred after the hypnosis. When we first met, she was suffering emotionally to the point the ship's crashing became her focal point in life. Now, she no longer cries every few minutes. She still talks about the ship's crashing, but no longer appears emotionally traumatized by it. She is more relaxed and talkative, as though a heavy burden has been removed.

It was interesting to note that prior to the hypnosis session in McKnight Canyon, Sanni walked with her shoulders slumped and would tire easily being out of breath after several minutes. After the session, with the removal of childhood traumas and the healing energies surrounding the retreat, she progressively began to walk in a more upright position and her energy continually increased.

Colette

"I was in my thirties when I went to visit my father, just a year before he died. He said, 'Do you know why you've had all these alien experiences since you were a baby, and UFO experiences, and why they've taken your babies from you?' I said, 'How did you know?' He said, 'I know, I just know,' and I responded, 'No, I don't know. Why?'"

Colette was a quiet, beautiful woman in her late forties with shoulder-length blonde hair and pale blue eyes the color of the sky on a sunny summer day.

She continued, "My father and mother were divorced since I was a child, and I don't ever recall telling my dad about these experiences. Then he said, 'You're a hybrid.' 'What do you mean, a hybrid?' I said. He responded, 'You're half human and half alien.' I said, 'You mean, Sophia and I are?' He said, 'No, only you.' I said, 'And Lydia?' and he said, 'No, only you.' I said, 'But I'm a twin.' He said, 'Colette, you are a hybrid. Sophia was an accident.'

"I didn't have much to do with my father for along time, and after he died, I began exploring this," she stated.

Needless to say, my curiosity was piqued, as I interjected, "You didn't find out how he knew?"

"No," Colette said, "but what was really weird, my father worked for the government, for the Army, and volunteered on some top-secret missions for the Army. We'd be gone for almost a year at a time. Nobody could know what was going on. A few years ago before my mother died, I asked her, 'Tell me how you got pregnant with Sophia and I.' My mother began, 'Well, that was the most peculiar thing I've ever experienced. You know Lydia was less than a year old, and your father was insistent that he didn't want any more kids at all. He'd been working as a bartender, then joined the army after Lydia was born because of the war. Strange thing was, the night I got pregnant with you girls, I came home and your dad was there with wine. That was unlike him. He said they were celebrating, but I didn't know what.' She said that she fixed dinner, then drank the wine and she said, 'I was drugged, like he put something in that wine. The next day, I didn't even remember that night and he said we had made love.' She said, 'That was so unlike him, because he would never have sex unless I had a diaphragm in, ever! And I don't remember a thing.' She said all of a sudden, when she was six or seven months pregnant, the doctor heard two heartbeats and said, 'Oh, you're going to have twins.' My mom said she was devastated because my sister wasn't very old. 'When you were born, Sophia was born in a sac like all fetuses are supposed to be, but you were not. The doctor couldn't find it.' Strangely enough, we had totally different blood types, and Sophia by the age of five was diagnosed with muscular dystrophy. She was so weak and I was so strong. I feel like I killed her.

"Since I was young, an extremely loving alien with golden eyes would appear to me while I was sleeping. He had wrinkly skin and three long fingers. He appeared as a spiritual teacher and would keep his eyes lowered in humbleness."

Colette wanted to be hypnotized to resolve the many questions she had from events in her lifetime, and to know more about this "loving alien."

After putting her into deep hypnosis, I regressed her back into her mother's womb.

D: Tell me what's going on.

C: I see myself with my eyes open, and I look at my little fist, and it looks odd.

D: Why does it look odd?

C: I see myself. My arms and legs look skinny.

D: Tell me what is going on.

C: I'm looking for Sophia.

D: Have you found her?

C: I don't think so.

D: Allow yourself to become younger, just after being in your mother's womb. As you are growing, tell me what's going on. Allow it to come into focus.

C: I seem to have freedom to move. I see Sophia, in a bubble, kind of a cocoon. But I'm not in a cocoon.

D: Ask your subconscious, why are you not in a cocoon?

C: There's like a tunnel, like something narrow. It's like I'm being put into something narrow. Oh! It's like being a, it reminds me of a wormhole.

D: Continue to follow it. Allow it to unfold in detail.

C: I see someone in a white smock. Very white skin. I'm not sure what I'm seeing.

D: Allow it to come forward. You can analyze it later.

C: This person I see has a very big head, very slender arms, very small neck, very skinny neck, very big eyes. Not human. I need to see the person better.

D: Allow it to come into focus, allow it to become clear.

C: (Sigh.) I see somebody standing beside this being. He's got a uniform on. Like a – some kind of a service uniform, looks like a tan color. I see military-like brass. It seems like this someone, this military man is observing, and – he's observing this being that was putting me in this tunnel, which I think is my mom. The being has a very, almost a light-bulb head.

D: Ask this being, does he have a name?

C: Jarars? I don't know, it sounds like Jara something. Jaras.

D: It's all right. Allow yourself to continue. Is there any relationship between you and this being, or is he just following orders?

C: I sense a feminine being. It's a female being, and I think she's just following orders.

D: Take a good look at yourself prior to being put in this tunnel, and describe what you see.

C: I'm in fluid. I seem to be like an – I don't know, like an itty-bitty spot in fluid. I don't know. It's like some kind of a, je – je – it's almost like a jelly, it's a thick, clear fluid, and, I just don't know, just a little spot.

D: Before you go into the tunnel, float around the area, and find out where the area is located.

C: Ooohhh – It looks like its some kind of – I get the feeling that the walls are brick or stone or something stone, the room I'm in.

D: This room that you are in. Is it on the earth plane or elsewhere?

C: I don't sense it's a UFO. I don't think it's a UFO. It seems like there's glass windows. Glass windows and people are observing through glass windows. I can't make out who's beyond there, other than I sense that there's people sitting and writing. I don't know why they're writing.

D: Go up and look at the paper and see what they're writing.

C: Well, it's not words. I don't know why, I'm getting symbols.

D: Just allow it to come forward. You can analyze it later. Do the people look like they're in human form or alien?

C: Alien.

D: Ask your subconscious. Are these the aliens that you came from? (Long pause.) What is the response?

C: I'm not getting anything.

D: Say goodbye to them. Allow yourself to be put into the tube. Now allow yourself to be put into your mother's uterus. See yourself growing larger and larger. Is there any information to come forth prior to being born?

C: I was just an experiment. I had no purpose.

D: Is it time to be born?

C: I see alien fingers around me. There are alien fingers around me. I don't know why. (Long pause.) I see my sister. And it's like she's in a cocoon. I don't understand why I can't touch her. I have freedom, but she doesn't.

D: Allow yourself to grow in size just prior to being born. If there is anything you need to know about your birth, allow it to come forward at this time.

C: I can't see myself being born. What I see, I'm not sure, it's almost like being sucked out.

D: Look around. Who is there during your birth?

C: I see a guy with glasses, white mask, umm, looks like he's wearing white clothes. He's an older man, probably middle-aged.

D: Is there anyone else?

C: Yeah, my mother, and there's a nurse. It's in a hospital.

D: Allow yourself to begin growing older. Go all the way to the original cause of feeling you killed your sister Sophia. Allow that to come into focus. Tell me in detail what is coming forward.

C: I feel like I was getting better nutrients, because I was free of the bubble, and I got more. It's like I got more nutrients.

D: You felt like you were getting more nutrients than Sophia causing her to not grow healthy. Scan your body, how is that making you feel?

C: She's just this little cupie doll, and I feel like, she's just a little baby and I'm more than a baby, like I've got more energy. I feel like – I feel strong, and she's just, seems like a little baby. I don't feel like a baby. I feel like a, I don't know. I observe her as a baby.

D: Is that causing any negative emotions within you physically, emotionally, or mentally?

C: I'm curious.

D: Go into that curiosity. Where are you holding onto that curiosity? Scan your body, where are you holding onto that curiosity of you being stronger and her being a baby?

C: I don't feel like I'm like her. I just feel like I'm – I don't know. I feel more like a person in a little body and I look at her as being interesting. I'm curious about her, but I don't think I'm aware that she's there, and that she's cute.

D: The feeling that you are stronger than her, and her being weaker than you, is that causing any distress within your physical form?

C: No. I kind of feel mothering in a way, and – I don't know, I can't quite feel it. I can't quite see it. I don't know. I just keep seeing this baby, before birth.

D: Would you like to hold this little baby before you leave, and comfort the little baby?

C: I want to touch it, and I want to look at it and see what it is.

D: Then allow yourself to do so; knowing you will be gentle.

C: I'm really curious because I don't understand why she's in this cocoon.

D: Look around; touch her.

C: I'd like to, but there's this bubble, like a bubble, a cocoon, but it's a clear bubble around her, and all I see is her shape. I keep wanting to take the bubble – open the bubble and see what's inside.

D: If you were to do that, would it harm what is inside?

C: Yeah. I'm just curious, but I don't feel alone.

D: Is it time to leave?

C: Yeah.

D: Then allow yourself to leave, going into the universe, the beauty of the stars, gently floating back and forth at peace, as you go down deeper and deeper and deeper. I ask now if you would like your father to come to you so that he may explain in more detail how you occurred, how he was aware. Would you like him to come forward?

C: Yes.

D: Then ask him to come forward and be here with you. Allow him to come forward. Is he here now? Allow the information to come into you, so you may have an understanding. Tell me what is going on.

C: I'm asking him why I was brought here. I see him as a young, young man. You know, I don't think that he cared. I don't think it was special. I think he just agreed to let me come. He agreed to let me be here. But it wasn't what he wanted. I don't know why, I'm sensing that he felt failure.

D: Why failure?

C: I feel that he was disappointed in Sophia. Mostly when she was younger, when she was a toddler. He expected more out of me, but (long pause.)

D: Is there any more information to come forward?

C: No.

D: Is there anything you would like to say to him before he leaves?

C: No.

D: There was an extremely loving alien with golden eyes from your past. He was a spiritual teacher, wrinkly skin, three long fingers. He would keep his eyes lowered in humbleness. Would you like him to come forward and be here with you?

C: Yeah.

D: Then ask him to come forward to be here and join you once again. Has he come forward?

C: Yes, I miss him.

D: What would you like to tell him?

C: To take me with him.

D: What is his response?

C: No. Things to do.

D: What are the things you have to do?

C: There are people. I have to help people.

D: Help them in what way?

C: I have to help people open their hearts and accept us, accept us all. We're all one!

D: How can you help people open their hearts and accept all of you?

C: Talk to them. Love them. And me, to teach them not to be afraid; help them through transition. I must be strong.

D: Is there any more information?

C: I must teach people not to be afraid, not to be afraid of us. It's like going to another – going someplace. Going to another world, so they're not afraid of this other world. It doesn't matter what we look like, if they understand that we're all inter-connected. I have to be more patient. I think I've forgotten who I am. I think I'm allowed to be human. I've forgotten why I am human.

D: Then allow that to come forward at this time. Why are you allowed to be human?

C: (Deep sigh.) For the transition. To help others into another – another something. It's like this ball, another formation, and it's like we're all going to go into this – I don't know. It's almost like another dimension, and it's pink, it's pink. Pink represents love. (Long pause.)

D: Allow yourself to continue.

C: Oh! I see myself as this white little alien, and my mentor is not like me. I'm white, and I'm like this creamy – like a ghost, because I'm. Oh! I don't have arms and legs or a body like humans. I see myself as looking almost – I don't see a body structure, I just see myself as being very thin, very skinny arms, skinny legs (deep sigh). I see a little belly on me, but I have this BIG head and a funny looking chin. It's not really a chin, it's like these wrinkles, and I have black eyes. I'm very white, and I have, I guess you could say, I almost look like a cartoon character because my fingers and toes are white, everything's stubby. I don't see any form. I don't see fingernails on me. (Pause.) I really don't like the way I look. I'm really disappointed because I certainly don't look human.

D: Feel your energy. Feel your inner energy of yourself. And now what comes forward?

C: I'm very loving. I'm innocent. I'm non-judgmental. I accept all things for what they are. I'm curious, and I feel like I'm burning up.

D: Burning up in what way?

C: I feel like I'm having a hot flash; I feel like I'm on fire.

D: Imagine cool, clear water. Allow yourself to cool down, cool clear water coming over you, washing over you, cleansing you, allowing the water to flow from the top of your head throughout your body, flowing out your toes, cooling (she interrupts.)

C: I look different now!

D: And now how do you look?

C: I've got more human features, but I'm still white. I've got little tiny features. I have a rounded head. That's interesting.

D: Is this as you were growing up?

C: No.

D: Is this as you were evolving?

C: Yeah. Yeah, I'm very irrides – no – what's the word? I'm not (pause).

D: Translucent?

C: Yeah, I'm not solid, but I have blue eyes, and a little, biddy nose, and I'm still a little white character, with round cheeks. I'm very humanoid looking, but I don't have any hair. Wow! I don't know how to explain me.

D: Allow it to come into focus within your brain, within your mind's eye, so that if you should wish to, you may do a sculpture of yourself.

C: (Begins crying.)

D: And now, do you feel the love for yourself?

C: (Crying louder.) Yeah.

D: Allow that love to grow stronger and stronger, knowing who you truly are and where you come from, and your true inner self. Allow the beauty, the innocent child, all those feelings to grow stronger within.

C: I come from a crystal world! (Crying harder, then calms down.) The world is crystal. It's blue crystals, white and blue. It's kind of like a whitish blue, and everything is like peaks, and it's a beautiful world. It doesn't have trees or anything though. It's like being on a crystal.

D: Is there a name for the crystal world that you come from?

C: It's almost see-through. It's like in a dimension that is not physical, as we know it, and it's like a crystal. Wow! It's like a globe, a crystal ball, and very innocent world. But it's – I just know that when I cooled off in the water, I transformed into this being that isn't physical or spiritual, but has shape, and of the Light. It's of the Light.

D: Are there any other forms from that world, from your world, any other human form that you now know of in your current lifetime that are also from your world? Allow them to come into focus.

C: (Deep sigh.) You're from that world. But you're from – you're higher! A Higher Light being, and that's why you're here! You're very, very special, that's why you're here. Wow! That's interesting. It's like a world – it's not a world! It's a pure form. Wow! I think we have to be trained and taught to be human. Why? What do we have to teach, be taught to be human? You would like the way we look. It's really nice, we don't have wings though, but we're of the Light. We're of the Light, and crystal. We are crystal. We appear, but we have to learn to be human, I think to teach others. Wow! We're here to teach others how to evolve. Maybe that's why I don't like being human, because I don't think humans are evolved. But you'd like what we look like, almost an iridescent pearl. How pretty! I think I understand that we have to go and experience, experience different lives. But with experience, there's pain. And

I don't like the pain. Maybe we all come from that. We all come from this place. (Long pause.) I'm ready to move on.

D: Thank them for showing you where you came from. Are you ready now to search further or are you ready to come out of hypnosis?

C: I'm ready to come out.

(Colette was taken to a peaceful place to re-energize and rest before coming out.)

Discussion after:

C: Our bodies are like a crystal, that look almost pearlish like a crystal, and unbelievable. I'll have to sculpture this. What I saw were deep, real sharp-like crystals. It was like where we're from is a dimension, all crystals around, and the crystals represent energy and love. When you asked me to cool down, I imagined getting into a blue lake of water, and when I did that, I took on this other form.

We're brought here, wow! This is part of how we learn. That was interesting. Our color is so much our bodies and our bodies are so much like crystal. Our bodies look like crystal, but yet we're not a solid form. Then again if you could see our heads and our faces, our faces are so angelic. Is it that we have all these things to learn before we go back?

D: We keep evolving, learning, and at the same time we're helping others learn and evolve. Maybe part of our growth is also helping others to grow.

C: The only thing I can think of is that being extraterrestrial, I required more nutrients and drank more nutrients that Sophia didn't get. I required more than her. She was diagnosed with muscular dystrophy, but her diagnosis didn't fit it completely. Her muscles never developed, yet I was born with incredible muscle tissue. As I was growing up and found out about this, I felt guilty for a long time and thought I had killed my sister.

She was only twenty-nine when she died. I remember being taken in the middle of the night by these people, it seemed like army nurses, and I was being taken to a facility below the floor. We came in on the ground level and this elevator went down so deep and it terrified me as a child because I didn't know where I was going, and this went on forever and ever down. I remember every time I cried they would tell me, don't cry. NO crying allowed. Don't speak. They were constantly testing me. I remembered my head and feet had to be covered up. I was always being taken by my feet by what I thought were little creatures. (As she continued to talk, the subject changed.) Growing up, I sat one time with my legs folded on the ground and talked to a snake and calmed the snake while the firemen were coming to get it. It was a diamondback rattler. I can do that but I can't explain it.

Colette told me several more stories where she was able to heal wounded animals and birds. She continued:

C: I didn't know plants had a life force. My husband has many rare plants. One of his rare plants, one of the hardest to grow, was rotted. He was trying to re-root it, and every so often I would check it. The rot was moving up, so I would cut more off. One day I picked it up, holding it in my arms, saying why can't I have powers to heal this, and all of a sudden I felt the pain of the plant. It went from one arm throughout my body and out the other arm. It was like I was being electrified because the pain was that strong. The vibration was incredible because of its pain.

Also, when I would walk past a plant and I would get really thirsty, I would turn around and look at the plant and know which plant needed water.

D: Maybe talking to and helping heal animals is the direction you need to be going in. You have an incredible connection with animals and plants. You have that gift within and now it's up to you if you choose to bring it forth to help others.

Colette did not come to me to remove emotional or mental pain, but to answer questions that had been plaguing her for many years. She relayed to me numerous extraterrestrial experiences and visits over her lifetime and felt comfort in the fact she was being taken care of and someone was watching over her. She has an amazing gift of talking to and healing plants and animals, which I fully encourage her to expand upon.

JoAnne,

Your new Crystal being will help you have conscious encounters & teach you spiritual lessons to help you evolve into the New World. You have chosen this being because you resonate a very high spiritual frequency.

Keep in touch.

In the Light,

Love & Blessings Always,

Cynthia

TIBET

SAMUEL

A tall, handsome man stood in my doorway waiting for his appointment. I was taken aback by his stature and by his strong, confident demeanor. I reminded myself that he had requested a hypnosis session because of his pull towards Tibet, not from any emotional problem or trauma he was seeking to uncover.

After regressing him, he was guided back to a lifetime in Tibet. He saw himself as a male, maybe ten years old, in the year "seventeen something."

S: (Deep breathing.) There seems to be a lot of people around. It seems to be a colder temperature, wearing clothes that are warm, cold-temperature oriented. There's not, I don't see snow.

D: Imagine looking down at your feet and tell me what you see.

S: It's like some sort of fur type, it's kind of like a boot, but it's like, it's got fur on it.

D: Allow yourself to look up. What are you wearing?

S: It's like a bulky kind of coat, fur hat.

D: Look around. Allow yourself to move forward to a significant event, and allow it to unfold in detail. Tell me what's going on.

S: Procession – a procession at the temple, the palace. I see yellow, elaborate robes, yellow, reds. I can hear the sounds of the hymns.

D: Who are wearing the robes?

S: They're the monks of the palace, coronation.

D: Coronation of who?
S: (Begins moving fingers.)
D: Tell me what's happening.
S: It's a, it feels like it's my father?
D: Is it the coronation of your father in that lifetime?
S: (Whispers.) Yes.
D: What is he called? What is his name?
S: (Gently sobbing, sniffing.) Rinpoche. It is His Holiness Rinpoche.
D: Allow the coronation to move forth. Tell me what's going on.
S: The procession is moving to the temple. It's a whole line, the procession. (Deep breathing.) They're wearing the big hats – they're monks – like brushes, yellow and reds, and His Holiness is seated in an elevated area with lots of yellow and reds, tapestries.
D: How is this making you feel as you watch the procession of your father, His Holiness?
S: It's an emotional time. He is the Father to all.
D: Allow yourself now to continue forth in that lifetime to another significant event and allow it to unfold in detail. Tell me what is going on.
S: My head is being shaved.
D: How old are you now?
S: Twelve.
D: Why is your head being shaved?
S: I am becoming a part of the Order. I have been taken in as have many children of my age, to study and become a part of the Order.
D: How does that make you feel?
S: (In a whining voice,) I don't like having my head shaved, but it is my duty.

D: Continue forward to another significant event in that lifetime. Tell me what's going on.

S: I am in prayer, wearing deep, red robes. It is quiet there.

D: How old are you now?

S: Twenty something. (Long pause.)

D: Tell me what's going on.

S: It's not clear.

D I ask your subconscious and super conscious to help clear it up. (Pause.) Tell me what's going on.

S: I'm walking with His Holiness. It's not the same as before.

D: What do you mean it's not the same?

S: It's not the same person.

D: Allow it to unfold. Tell me what's going on.

S: I just see myself walking with His Holiness.

D: How are you dressed?

S: As a monk.

D: How old are you?

S: Middle twenties.

D: Move forward to a significant event. Let me know what is going on.

S: I feel like I'm high up. There's wind blowing around me. I can see the clouds above me.

D: What is the importance of this vision?

S: My arms are outstretched. The wind is blowing and my robes are blowing in the wind. The wind is really strong around me. (Takes a deep breath.)

D: Is this the same lifetime you've been in or is this a different dimension?

S: I am not touching the ground, although it is not far from my feet. I travel across the – there are others that are there watching me from the ground, which is not far away.

D: What allows you to travel and not touch the ground? What form are you in?

S: I am a person. I have learned to fly.

D: What year is it?

S: 18 something.

D: What land are you in?

S: I am in Lhasa.

D: Is it a knowing within?

S: Yes, as far as the means of being able to leave the ground is part of one's thought patterns, whereas we can manipulate the forces around us by tapping into the matrix. I get chills when I say it.

D: What is the significance of the chills?

S: It is the truth.

D: Allow yourself to continue bringing forth the information for your knowledge.

S: It is the tone and the breath which allows us to transcend gravity, dimension, allows us to travel.

D: How will this knowledge help you in your future?

S: It will allow me to travel above areas that do not permit me to physically touch the ground. It will allow me to see what is. It will allow me to lead others to safety.

D: Is this something you will use to teach others or use for yourself? Tell me what's going on.

S: I am still hovering and moving about the sky, above the people who I am working with, learning to manipulate objects as well, allowing them to move as I move. There's a great freedom to move about the sky, to be able to move freely, to manipulate objects with one's hands.

D: Is this knowledge you have brought forth into your current lifetime?

S: Yes.

D: Then allow it to become stronger within you. Allow yourself to understand the techniques and whatever is necessary. Allow it to be solidified within your consciousness in your current lifetime. Let me know when it is done.

S: It already has.

D: If it is not already in your consciousness, then go into your brain and see a switch. This is a switch, when it is time, you can turn the switch on and allow yourself to access all the information immediately, so that you may help others. Do you see the switch?

S: Yes.

D: Identify it however you choose so that when it is time, you may flip the switch and all the information will be readily accessible within your consciousness, so that you will be able to do whatever is necessary to help others in your current lifetime. Is that agreeable?

S: Yes.

(It was indicated earlier, but not included, that Sam had lived many lifetimes in Tibet.)

D: Then allow it to be so. Now, looking over all the lifetimes in Tibet with His Holiness when you gained knowledge, is there any more information you need to bring forth into your current knowledge that will help you in the work that you will be doing in your current lifetime? Allow the information to come forth.

S: I'm in a class. They are teaching us how to travel in a different manner than before. The instructor dematerializes and reappears in the other part of the room. It's a means of travel. He says we are capable of traveling great distances by using our own abilities within us, by tapping into the source, with proper tone and breath.

D: Bring forth those tones and breaths within yourself so you have the knowledge in your current lifetime and can access them when necessary. Allow them to come forth. (Pause.) Are you now aware of the tones?

S: They are there, but I have not grasped them, but they are there. I'm getting chills again.

D: What is necessary for you to grasp them?

S: To release the control of self.

D: Is it time to release the control of self?

S: No, but soon.

D: Will you know when the time will come?

S: Yes.

D: Is that a knowing within yourself?

S: Yes.

D: Then allow the tones to come forth within yourself when it is time. Is that agreeable?

S: Yes.

D: Is there any more information to come forth to your current lifetime?

S: There is a seer. He is bringing forth information for His Holiness. There are many around him because he goes through convulsions. He is like all over the place, and they attempt to restrain him. He is heavily ornamented in ceremonial-type robes and headdress.

D: What is the importance of the seer being there for you?

S: The ending of our way of life. We can no longer walk free. We are told the Chinese are coming. (Long pause, becoming emotional.) They – destruction, the killings (shivers) that we must go.

D: Where must you go?

S: We must leave the city.

D: Allow yourself to move forth. As you leave the city, tell me what's happening.

S: Chaos.

D: What year is it now?

S: 19 something.

D: Move forward, just prior to passing over in that lifetime, just prior to your death. Tell me what's going on.

S: We are being shot down. (Becoming very emotional.) It is a mass of gunfire as we are gathered together. (Whispers.) We are all killed.

D: Scan your body. Is there pain caused from being shot down still within your physical body?

S: I believe there is a trace memory of it still.

D: Where is it in your physical body?

S: It doesn't feel like a specific place in my body, other than the trauma of the occurrence because it was done so quickly.

D: Then imagine pulling off that trace within yourself and throwing it back on them. Is there is anything you would like to tell them, allow yourself to do so. What would you like to tell them?

S: They are forgiven. (Long pause.)

D: Where are you now?

S: I'm with my people.

D: Who are your people?

S: They are from Sirius.

D: What information would they like to share with you?

S: There are others. There's a gathering. There are those that are not from this planet, but I know them. There is a council from many different universes. I have been chosen to be a messenger, to travel to many worlds, to talk of peace, to learn the ways of many, to show others how very much like them other people's beings are, that we need to work together to preserve that which we are. There have been some appointed personnel that monitor me, my progression, in this particular divisional plane. It is different here than other places; they do not understand here. The people here are logical, they are curious. They have come here to do as I, to observe, and to assist when the time comes. This is a place of gathering, this place in which we live.

D: What do you mean by gathering?

S: We are here to create a matrix, that which will preserve the species as we move into another plane. Many will transcend, but many will not, and that is the way it is to be. Everything is changing; time, space, it affects us all. I am here because I am known by many. They recognize me, not as a physical being but as a vibrational being. I've been here for a long time and I'm tired. You are one of many who stayed behind when the rest were taken away. There was a period when many were removed from the planet; many of us chose to stay. Civilizations disappeared abruptly. It was when they returned from whence they came, but many of us chose to stay behind to work on the planet and the beings that remained here in an attempt to populate a species that was moonlight-oriented, because they became corrupted. And now we are here once more to do it again. This is my last time here, for I no longer choose to remain. And when the time comes, I shall be removed, but the time seems so far off.

Many who we associate with now are part of the group that was here before. We gather information, we connect with different people as they pass through who respond to our vibration and not know why, but we give them information in different ways that act as keys to the openings of their memories. That is why people come and go from our lives so quickly, because they come to us for the key to unlock the memories to go on and do what they must do, whether they are conscious of it or not. Sometimes just our touch will alter their vibration. We gather together because we are familiar and over the millennia of time, the familiarity is a comfort. But there is much to do, as time grows short. But there is no need to fear of what is to come for we have experienced it before. It is just a thought. There is much to prepare for, but there is very little to do.

D: How shall we prepare?

S: By being clear, not living in the fear of the masses around us. It is so hard to separate from the consciousness here. It causes us to lose our way.

D: Are you on your correct path for your destiny?

S: We are all where we should be at a particular time, so when the time comes our memory access will be activated fully, and those who wish to do what they're here for, will do so. Should they pick otherwise, it is their choice. But many shall do what they set out to do. That's why we're here and why we were chosen, 'cause ultimately we would know that we would do what is right. This is an odd world we live in. It is so full of deception. It is full of beauty, but yet we tear it apart. We destroy everything we touch in this world, and yet they think they are doing it for some higher purpose, which there's no (becomes emotional.) There is much to prepare, yet there is nothing to prepare, for what is this? So many people fear what is to come. There is nothing to fear, for it is. Everyone shall be where they should be and do what they elected to do. There is no need for fear. Fear is what you must fear, for in fear you are in darkness, without it, you see things clearly and you know what to do. You don't allow your emotions to take control over you, and you act appropriately in the situation because there is no place to run to, for all will be affected, some more seriously than others. And those that transcend during certain periods, it is nothing to be fearful of, for they chose to leave this world in that manner, for the physical body is only a vehicle. It is our essence self which lives on for millennia of time as we grow and evolve and become non-physical. In doing so, we have the ability to move from place to place easily without constraints, without outside vehicles.

Humans give so much to others. They rely on everything to do what they themselves can do, for they've become lazy and have forgotten who they are. But they shall remember soon. And those that are here to corrupt those who are here to help, they will not gain foothold this time for although they shall continue to cause strife, their days here are limited for the changes were close at hand before, but those who wish to manipulate did so. They caused it to continue, but the time has come for more changes and this time they will not be allowed for consciousness wants change. They are tired of the old ways and it's time to move on.

D: Before you leave your people from Sirius, is there any information they would like to give you personally?

S: I know that they are always with me.

End of session.

After bringing Sam out of hypnosis, he said he had a dull headache, "like a tightness in the head." After a few moments, the headache disappeared. He was given a taped copy of his hypnosis session as he left. Several days later, I called to see how he was doing. He said each time he listened to the tape, during a particular part in the tape his headache returned. I requested he come in to see me again.

The following week, Sam came to my office. I suggested he be regressed to a time in Tibet again to find the cause of his headaches. He agreed.

After being regressed, he saw himself standing in heavy fur boots, animal skins for his coat, and a large furry hat, looking into the distant mountains. He wasn't sure of his age, just that he was, "Not a child, but I'm not old either."

D: Now as you stand overlooking the mountains in the foreground, why are you standing where you are?

S: I seem to be tending my livestock.

D: What is your livestock?

S: I have a yak.

D: What is the feeling that surrounds you as you tend your yak?

S: Just an average day. Nothing particular. Doing my chores.

D: Allow yourself now to move forward to an important time within that lifetime, to an important event. Allow it to unfold.

S: There seems to be some strange visitors.

D: In what manner are the visitors strange?

S: They're not from here.

D: Where are they from?

S: I believe they come from Orion.

D: Why have the visitors come forth?

S: I'm not sure why they're here.

D: Ask them why they're there. Are they there to visit Tibet or are they there to specifically visit you?

S: They are here for some others and me. I remember seeing them before. I remember seeing something in the sky before when I was out with my animals. I thought it was a strange thing and now, they are here. Strange looking.

D: Would you like to describe them?

S: They seem to be very skinny and I don't know why they're not cold because they're not wearing warm clothes. I don't know what they're wearing. They don't seem to be wearing much of anything, but it's hard to describe. It's like they're wearing nothing, but they must be wearing something. They seem to want to take us with them.

D: Do they take you with them?

S: I feel like I'm going with them with some other boys. They want to show us something, but I don't know why.

D: Allow them to show you. Allow it to unfold.

S: No one seems to think it's strange that we're going. It seems that people watch us going, but no one says anything. I don't seem to be that old. No one else seems to be that old, but they're taking us.

D: Where are they taking you?

S: In that thing they're flying. Big inside. Some of the boys are afraid.

D: How do you feel at that time?

S: Curious, but I'm not afraid. They're taking us inside and we're walking through and there are others inside. Big – very unusual things that we don't have.

D: Would you like to describe the things or is it unimportant.

S: (Voice becomes childlike.) They just look like things. It seems as though there's something that they're putting the boys into. It's like they're locking them in something.

D: What is the reason for this?

S: I'm not sure.

D: What is happening to you?

S: They're taking me to a different area. The rest of the boys have been locked in something.

D: Allow them to take you to the different area and tell me what happens.

S: They seem to be interested in me, different from the others.

D: Why are they interested in you, different from the others?

S: I don't know why they think I'm different.

D: Ask them. Why do they think you're different?

S: They say I'm chosen for something.

D: What are you chosen for?

S: They want to know why I can do things.

D: What do you tell them?

S: I don't know. I just do. They want to examine me closely. (Takes a deep breath.) The other boys don't seem to be, there's something going on with them. They're yelling. I don't know what they're doing to the other boys, but it doesn't feel right.

D: How does that make you feel?

S: A little uncomfortable. They tell me not to listen, not to worry. It does not concern me. But it does concern me.

D: Where are you holding onto that concern? Where is the cause of that concern within you?

S: Here, (rubs chest) it seems like something. It doesn't feel like, they want to check me out further. They have things that keep me from going anywhere.

D: What do you mean by that? Are you in restraints?

S: Yeah. I'm not sure what they want to do, but the other boys are frightened. I'm not sure what they're doing, but they're very frightened. It makes me a little concerned.

D: Allow it to unfold and continue. What do they do to you?

S: They're examining me.

D: How are they examining you?

S: They're examining my head and looking into my eyes and mouth and doing something. It feels weird.

D: What are they doing and where are they doing it?

S: It's around my head. It's like this thing they put around my head. They said they want to monitor my brain.

D: Describe what they put around your head.

S: It's kind of like a big hat, but it's, I don't know what it's made of, something like metal.

D: How is that making your head feel?

S: I don't really feel anything. It's just that I don't like it around my head, and the boys keep yelling. I don't know why. They're not hurting me, but I don't know why everyone else is having a problem.

D: Do they keep this metal hat around your head indefinitely or do they remove it?

S: They take it off after a while.

D: Has this caused any pressure within your brain?

S: I don't feel funny. I just don't know what it is they're trying to figure out. I don't know why they think I'm different from everyone else.

D: Ask your subconscious, your Higher Self, is this knowledge that will help you to have the unfolding of the events?

S: I feel like, that whatever it is that they feel that I can do will become stronger when I get big, because I can see things and I can do things, but I don't know why they think it's different.

D: Is there anything else within that immediate time frame that needs to come forth for you to view?

S: The boys don't come with me when they let me go.

D: How does that make you feel?

S: I don't know why they don't let them go.

D: What is that causing within your mind?

S: It really upsets me because they were yelling and then they wouldn't let them go.

D: Is that causing pressure within your brain, within your head?

S: (Deep breath.) No. I don't think so.

D: Go into your chest area. Has that become heavier because of the yelling of the boys and their not coming back with you?

S: (Pause.) I don't feel like I have anything the matter with me.

D: Allow yourself now to fast forward to when you become older, to another important event within that lifetime, one that has caused headaches to occur from the remembrance of it. Allow it to come forward and unfold in detail. Tell me what is going on.

S: I'm doing things. I'm able to move things without touching them. The monks work with me. I've worked with objects floating around and I'm able to fly, too. It just seems like the more I do stuff, my head does feel pressure at times.

D: Go into that pressure. Find the cause that is creating the pressure within your head. Walk around your brain and find the cause.

S: I feel like it's because there's so much energy coming through my head, that it's very – sometimes it – they want me to do too much.

D: Who are they?

S: Those that I work with. It is almost like they want me to go beyond what I'm doing. It's like I'm being pressured to do more.

D: Who are you referring to when you say those who you are working with?

S: It is the members of our Order.

D: Do you mean the monks?

S: Yes. And there are others that also are observing, like those that were here before and different ones.

D: Go up to them and ask them, have they been helping you to excel in your gifts?

S: They're encouraging me to develop it further because they know I can do more. They feel I have it within me. It is something that I have always been able to do and they don't know what makes me different from everyone else, but I'm able to do things and they want me to do more.

D: And that is causing you pressure in your head?

S: Yeah, because I don't want to do it all the time.

D: Go into your head. Ask your subconscious and your super conscious, is it time to release some of that pressure in your head from the memory of that lifetime?

S: No. It's important that I know how to do these things.

D: But do you have to have the pressure in your head in order to know how to do them?

S: No!

D: Then allow yourself to release some of that pressure. You can retain the gifts, but you no longer need to have the pressure. Imagine with your third eye, imagine it opening and releasing some of that pressure, retain all your gifts, but releasing some of the pressure that has been caused by that energy. Allow it to come out like the opening of a balloon, releasing some of the pressure. Feel it coming out your third eye. (Pause.) Tell me what's going on.

S: They don't like it when I resist them. They try to make me work harder and do things that cause my head to hurt.

D: What type of things do they do to cause your head to hurt?

S: They do it with their minds. They want me to push harder and I don't want to push harder. I know I can do things, but they want me to do them all the time.

D: By they, do you mean the beings from Orion?

S: Yes, and the other ones. They say it's important that I know these things. They want to see how extensive my abilities are because they know there is much that I can do, and they want to learn from it. They want to know why I can do it and how I can teach others to be that way because many of them have abilities as well, but my abilities are different. They have no real feelings, but I do and that's a curiosity. They tell me I've always had these things; that I'm not really from there.

D: Where are you from?

S: They say I originate from Sirius B, what is known as Sirius B, that system. I was taken from there when I was very young and seeded here and raised by these people. My family had these abilities and they were feared.

D: By your family, do you mean your family in that lifetime in human form?

S: No, my family who bore me.

D: What are they called?

S: (Deep breath.) Bor, Bora. It's a name that comes to me, I'm not sure why. There were a lot of problems in my world and that's why I was removed, because I was different. At the time I was born, I was different. I do not know why, but I was taken from my family and seeded here.

D: Seeded where?

S: In Tibet. I was raised here. But those that bore me did not come from here, but I was raised here and I was kept away from others so it would not interfere with my development until it was time. I was inducted into the Order when I became of age, because even then I was doing things, and they wanted to observe me closely. And so, I was put within the Order so I could be monitored closely without the interference from the outside. There was always a lot of pressure put on me to develop, but I didn't want to. I knew I could, but there were always things; they didn't want to leave me alone. And sometimes my head would hurt because they always wanted me to study so hard.

D: They were doing this for your benefit and your growth. As a young child you were not aware of that. As an adult, did you become more aware of that?

S: I knew that I was being prepared to do things because I learned to do many things here and I showed them how to do things as well, and how easy it was to do things. I felt that, I don't feel people were afraid of me because I never gave them a reason to be afraid. I just seemed to do well with some people, although some of the people that would come from other places, I did not like.

D: Why did you not like them?

S: They weren't nice to people.

D: In what way?

S: They, (deep breath) the reptile people I didn't like. They made me uncomfortable. I've never felt comfortable with the reptilian people. They were from that place before when I was little, but I didn't notice them that much then. They looked different.

D: What was their energy like?

S: They wanted me to do things that were bad. They wanted me to hurt people and I don't do that. I didn't want to do that and they couldn't make me do that. The other people were better and there were a lot of different people that came. They would monitor me when I got older, two people from my world.

D: How did they monitor you?

S: They would either come and visit me in person or they had ways of observing me from a distance.

D: Now, as you are older in that lifetime, how does your head feel? Do you still have pressure in your head from all your learning?

S: Maybe a little, but not like it had been before. I work closely with Kondune. He speaks with me often. (Voice changed as though beginning to cry.)

D: Who is Kondune?

S: He headed our Order. He is the Dalai Llama.

D: Is it acceptable to allow him to come in front of you and put his hands around your head, on your forehead, around your neck and your shoulders and release any pain or pressure that was caused by an excess of energies from your learning and excelling in that lifetime? Will you allow him to do this?

S: If he desires to do so.

D: Then I ask if he would desire to do so, would he lay his hands upon you to release excess energies that have caused pain and headache, pressure within your head. (Long pause.) Tell me what is happening.

S: (Sounding stuffed up.) I don't know why, I always feel so emotional around His Holiness.

D: It is the unconditional love that he generates, the unconditional love for you, that overwhelming feeling of love. Allow it to become part of you. Feel your body, your head, your neck, and your shoulders at peace, relaxed, with his love within you, at peace. (Long, deep breath coming from Sam.) And now, is there any more information from that lifetime to be brought forth that will help you in your current lifetime?

S: Yes.

D: Then allow it to come forth and tell me in detail what is going on.

S: I am to be taken from there when I transcend. My physical form is not to remain, but I will be removed at the proper time. When my time ends there, I will move on; part of me has already gone.

D: How old are you when that occurs?

S: I am old. It would seem that from there I was to work with the Council, the Council which is not of this world.

D: Is it time now to go to the Council?

S: Yes.

D: Allow yourself to go to the Council, to be in front of the Council. If it is permissible, allow the information to come forth.

S: I was chosen from an early age, from the time I was born, to work with the Council, to travel to other worlds and to find ways to have peace within the universe. There has been much unrest in certain sectors and the need for domination. It is no longer acceptable, and many among the ranks or those who wish to control are seeing that it is not necessary to do so. The reptilians are feared by many because they are brutal and in many cases consume those that defy them, consume both their resources as well as their physical beings. They are above the rat race. There are many that have formed alliances with them out of fear of destruction; even within the ranks there is unrest. They do not attempt to harm me, although there was a time that they did. I always must be careful in their sectors for they do not approve of what I am doing, for it is a way for them to no longer be the way they are.

I have traveled many places and have used my abilities to counsel, to heal, to have great strength, and not just as in physical strength for most of my energies come from within. My abilities are known throughout the different sectors, for they know I am able to travel at will and I am able to do many things for many people and to show them how they, too, can to do these things to better their lives and their worlds, and to use the abilities for peaceful means for the benefit for the good of all their people. I don't feel like I'm doing anything special, but I am well respected by many. And that is why I do the work that I'm doing because the others had seen that I was coming to be, and it is why I was nurtured even though I did not like it, being forced to use my abilities and bringing them forth when I was young. It was something that I needed to do. The times that I spent on the earth plane during that time period were important. I've lived dual lifetimes while there, as part of my growth and continue to do so. I'm also living simultaneously in other realms so that I may grow faster and do my work in more places at one time, at different levels, for it is my purpose.

Although there are some that wish to stop what I do, I am protected and I need not live in fear, although there are times when I do feel the discomfort of those who may come close, but I do not live in fear. But there are times when it is frustrating because I am limited until a certain stage to be able to utilize what I can do. But I must be careful when utilizing the abilities for it causes an uncomfortable feeling for others and the potential of being used by those who do not have your best interest at heart. And so I live a meager life until it is time for me to do what I came here to do.

I feel the time comes soon when I will better utilize my abilities for the benefit of many as we prepare for the shift. I am preparing many in many areas simultaneously for the shifting will occur, not just on the present planet on which this physical body now exists, but on all the many levels that work around it. And so at times I feel very drained because I am doing so much in so many places at this time, but it is what I do and why I am here. And I have been here for a long time, and it was my choice to do so for I was chosen to do it. It was my duty to do so; therefore I am.

Many are here at this time because it is an important time for all to develop rapidly during this vibrational period. Many tend to journey with those that are familiar with them so they may interact for comfort and growth. Fear holds us all back because when there is fear there is blockage. You do not think clearly, you do not act in a clear manner. These are interesting times that we live in and there is much more disruption to come and it will increase, but there is no reason to fear, for all shall be well. For we are only in the physical in this time space, and we will continue to work in this time space until it is time for us to go on. That which we are lives forever. The form that we have taken is just for the now.

D: Is there any more information to be brought forth before we end?

S: No. I feel this is all that is necessary at the present time.

End of session.

As Sam was coming out of hypnosis, he said, "Well, I don't have that pressure that I had last time. It seemed very different this time around. I'm really surprised about the ET's there. It's interesting."

As an added note, Sam decided to research his past and e-mailed me his findings. The following are his comments from the first hypnosis session:

I decided to investigate what I perceived during the original regression for my own verifications. I thought I would share my findings with you. The Rinpoche family lineage dates back to when Buddhism was first introduced to Tibet. They were spiritual teachers to the Dalai Lamas and acting Regents until the new Dalai came of age. As far as I can tell, the lineage starts with Phakchok Rinpoche and his incarnations and family that follow. Reting Rinpoche was Regent during the time of the 13th and 14th Dalais. His Holiness was born in 1935 and became the official ruling Dalai Lama at age 15 in 1950.

In the spring of 1959, he consulted the Nechung Oracle due to the increasing problem with the Chinese. The Oracle wore a huge headdress and heavy silk robes that could not be supported until the channeling began. He would then go into convulsions and run all over the place as the attendants attempted to restrain him. He instructed the Dalai to leave that night into exile due to the impending takeover of the Chinese forces. He was smuggled out of Lhasa and entered India in exile on March 31, 1959. Many atrocities took place in Tibet and many monks and civilians were brutally killed and tortured. It was the end of the old way of life for Tibet and its people. I think we were on track for the period. The robes worn by the Dalai and the monks were deep red and bright yellow. Headdresses were like brushes on their heads also in yellow. Tibetan Buddhism also incorporated Vajrayana or tantra into their teachings with an underlying influence of the White Bon religion that was prior to Buddhism. It deals with magic and metaphysical and the forces of nature. Pretty darn interesting!!!! I feel something will come of this regression experience. We shall see. Thanks Dr. D for your help in bringing this to light.

SUFFOCATION AND ABANDONMENT

CYNTHIA

Cynthia is her early forties. Although she has loving parents, she complained of feelings of abandonment, loneliness, and suffocation. She said she felt lost and wanted to try hypnosis to free herself of these inner feelings. The hypnosis began:

D: Go to the original cause of feeling like you're suffocating.

C: (Rubbing her neck.) Feels stiff, going to shoulders.

D: Go into what is causing your shoulders and neck to feel stiff.

C: There's a chain around my neck.

D: What are you wearing?

C: I don't know if I'm a slave. I don't know what I am, but I have a four-inch metal collar around my neck, chained behind me – I can't (pause.)

D: Imagine looking around. Is there anyone else around? Describe what you see.

C: It's flat. There's sand, flat, and there's like a large square-block building. I don't know if it's Egyptian or what. I don't know.

D: Imagine turning around and looking at yourself and describe what you see.

C: My skin is dark and I'm shiny, bald head.

D: Are you male or female?

C: Male.

D: How old are you?

C: Twenty-three, I think.

D: Allow yourself to become younger, prior to having the metal collar put around your neck. Tell me what's going on.

C: I'm young, thin, black.

D: Go to the scene just prior to having the metal collar put around your neck. What caused you to have the collar put around your neck?

C: I feel I'm alone, alone and younger. I'm kind of like squatting down. It's open. I don't see much around me other than just me.

D: Why are you squatting down?

C: I'm gathering something. I think I'm gathering something to eat. I'm not sure. I'm real thin. My head is large; my body is thin. Nobody's around me.

D: Go to a significant time just prior to the collar being put around your neck.

C: I'm alone. They look like herders, big game hunters. I look like a cartoon character in the aspects of the body and everything. None of it seems real.

D: Bring forth more information.

C: Because I was alone, because I was only one and there were no others, because I was different, I was unique, there are no others around me. It's almost like they didn't want to lose me, they didn't want me to go, so they had me bound so I wouldn't escape.

D: Go into the feelings of being unique. What feeling does that bring forth, unique?

C: Kind of lonely, having to take care of my own, having to find my own way of survival, no other sources to rely on other than what I found before me, not really having an understanding of what I'm here for.

D: Where is that coming from, not having an understanding of what you're here for?

C: I was just dropped off.

D: Go all the way back to when you were dropped off. Who dropped you off?

C: Like a satellite, I guess.

D: Go into the satellite.

C: It's a saucer, satellite-like.

D: Keep going into it. Who dropped you off? What was the reason you were dropped off?

C: I get the word observation.

D: Imagine turning around. Look at who has been observing you.

C: It was the gray from above the saucer, seeing how I'd fare and how the people would find me and what they would do to me.

D: Ask them now to come forth to you. What have their observations been? What were the results of dropping you off?

C: I get the word nothing.

D: Why nothing?

C: Didn't go as planned.

D: What was planned?

C: I don't get the picture, I don't know.

D: Just allow it to come forth. You can analyze it later. What did they have planned? What did they expect when they dropped you off?

C: I guess they expected me to do more.

D: Do more in what way?

C: Because I was just huddling over in a crouched position and stagnate. (Becomes agitated.) I don't know what they want!

D: Ask them. Allow it to come forth one word at a time. What did they want?

C: Me, to bring in people.

D: Bring in people. What do they mean?

C: (Begins yelling.) I don't know! I'm not getting anything! I'm dead!

D: Go back to the collar around your neck, back to the cause. Is it time to release the collar from around your neck?

C: No.
D: Why is the response no?
C: Restriction.
D: Why is it necessary to have restriction?
C: Holding back.
D: Why is it necessary to hold back?
C: Not time.
D: Not time for what?
C: Need more information. (Begins squirming in chair.)
D: (Loudly.) Tell me what's happening!
C: (Begins crying.) They just left me, gave up and left me. I'm frustrated and confused. I don't understand what my purpose is, why I'm here, dropped! I'm just left! I'm abandoned! And I have this around me and I have no one to turn to. I don't know what to do!
D: Go to that feeling of being abandoned. Where are you holding onto it within your body? Scan your body.
C: (Becoming calmer.) My gut.
D: Go into your gut. Imagine blowing up a balloon, completely enclosing the feeling of abandonment. If you were to give it a color, what color would it be?
C: A blue, a dark blue.
D: Begin pushing the dark blue balloon filled with abandonment down your leg out onto the floor, being grounded into Mother Earth. Keep pushing it out your leg. Where is it now?
C: In my left leg.
D: Keep pushing it out.
C: I can't!
D: Yes you can! Keep pushing it out. I ask your grandpa to come in and give you extra strength. (During the intake, she stated she was very close to her grandpa and grandma who had passed over several years earlier.) Keep pushing it out. Is your grandpa with you now?

C: (Crying.) My grandma.

(Many of those on the spirit side are here to help us. Under hypnosis, a person can interact with a deceased loved one for several reasons. It may be to feel their love once more, finish unresolved issues, or to give the client strength. He or she may need help to face and remove a problem that has caused energy blocks that the client does not feel strong enough emotionally to handle alone.)

D: Keep pushing. She's helping you. She's with you. Keep pushing it. Where is it now?

C: (Gently sobbing.) Ankle.

D: Keep pushing. She's smiling as she's helping you. She's giving you her love and her strength to keep pushing it.

C: (Deep breaths, becoming softer.) I'm trying to get it out. This leg's fine, (grabbing her right leg), but my left leg's still a little dark; it seems dark.

D: Go into the darkness, all the way into the darkness, to the cause.

C: The ship is gone, having to fend for myself in an area that I don't know where I am, how to deal with it, and I feel helpless.

D: In the area of the darkness in your leg, can we add bright light, and the love of your grandma to that area? Will that help lighten it and brighten it?

C: Yes.

D: Then allow that area of your leg to become brighter and brighter with your grandma's love. Feel her energy, knowing she is with you. You no longer are alone. She is with you. Your leg is becoming lighter and brighter, removing the loneliness, replacing it with her love. Let me know when you have finished.

C: It's gone; it's light.

D: Let's go back into the abdomen, where you have removed the feelings of abandonment. What would you like to fill it with?

C: Security.

D: What color would security be for you?

C: Gold.

D: Then allow yourself to fill the entire area in your abdomen with the color gold, representing security. Let me know when you have completed this.

C: I'm done.

D: Go back to the time just prior to your passing, with the large metal collar around your neck. Imagine shrinking yourself, slipping out of the collar, and going back to the clasp of the collar. Reach (she interrupted.)

C: I, myself, vanished. I disintegrated into sand before I ever got to the clasp. The clasp was in the back of my neck and I disintegrated.

D: You disintegrated and the clasp is no longer around your neck.

C: I disintegrated. I am no longer.

D: You are no longer, so the clasp is empty?

C: The clasp is sitting there on the ridge. It was like a table. I was standing up, but it was like, chained back.

D: The clasp is no longer around your neck because you have disintegrated.

C: I disintegrated in my head and I disintegrated out of it, like the sand in the hourglass.

D: Imaging healing your neck. Allow yourself to send healing golden rays, golden energy to your neck, healing your neck from where the clasp was suffocating it. Allow your neck to become stronger, to feel free. Allow yourself to be able to breathe freely once again. Feel the freedom from within. It feels good.

C: (Takes deep breath, and releases it slowly.)

End of session.

~ ~ ~

In Cynthia's regression, she saw herself as an alien, confused after being dropped off from a saucer. As with Sanni, it is not for me to believe or discount as a fantasy what Cynthia experienced. The issues here that her subconscious brought forth are emotional scars of abandonment, suffocation, and loneliness, which she was able to remove so she can move forward in her current lifetime without unnecessary obstacles in her way. Cynthia has since called me, telling me of great strides in her relationship with her boyfriend, no longer thinking or feeling he is going to leave her. She also said she can wear close-fitting collars around her neck without panicking, something she was unable to do in the past.

Chapter 7

The Other Side of the Veil

Are you afraid of death? Do you wonder what is going to happen to you after you die? Is it possible you have a spirit, which came from somewhere else and will return there after your body dies, or is this just wishful thinking because you are afraid? These are questions brought forth by Michael Newton, Ph.D., in his book, *Journey of Souls, Case Studies of Life Between Lives*. He spent many years researching life in the spirit world. He continues:

> If death were the end of everything about us, then life indeed would be meaningless. However, some power within us enables humans to conceive of a hereafter and to sense a connection to a higher power and even an eternal soul. If we do actually have a soul, then where does it go after death? The true answers to the mystery of life after death remain locked behind a spiritual door for most people. This is because we have built-in amnesia about our soul identity, which, on a conscious level, aids in the merging of the soul and human brain.

For those who have had the opportunity to actually see their immortality, a new depth of self-understanding and empowerment emerges. Having a conscious knowledge of their soul life in the spirit world and a history of physical existences on planets gives these people a stronger sense of direction and energy for life. Thoughts about the spirit world involve universal truths among the souls of people living on Earth.

As a hypnotherapist, when I feel it will benefit the client, I ask if they would like to go "behind the veil." By this I mean taking them to the time prior to being in their mother's womb. Information gleaned from this type of hypnosis helps them understand and accept many of the events that have happened to them. They receive information from the subconscious or superconscious as to why they may have been plagued with illness or physical deformity throughout their lifetime, along with many other insights, which gives them an understanding of their physical traits along with other revelations, and they come back with an acceptance of themselves.

Sarnie

Sarnie is a lovely woman in her early sixties, a gifted astrologer and psychic. When she first came to my office, several months earlier she had been operated on for the removal of cancer from her body. She was now in the process of having chemotherapy. Much of her life has been wrought with sudden illnesses. Through her years, she had been operated on numerous times. Some of the operations were planned, yet others were unexpected. After working with Sarnie on several occasions via hypnosis, we both decided it was time to go to the "other side of the veil" for further information.

Sarnie has been age-regressed, and is now in her mother's womb:

D: How are you feeling?

S: I'm uncomfortable. My skin itches. It stings a little bit.

D: Ask your subconscious, what is causing the itching?

S: It's toxicity, I can hear a big heartbeat.

D: What is the toxicity doing to you at this stage of your growth?

S: It's just irritating.

D: Listen to your parents talking. How are they feeling about you?

S: Very excited, but worried.

D: Why are they worried?

S: Money. They need to move; they need more space, and they're worried about having the money.

D: Do you have any reaction to this after you are born?

S: No.

D: Is there any more information for you in the embryo stage?

S: They worry too much about money. They don't need to.

(At this point, I regressed Sarnie into her most recent past lifetime.)

S: I'm in a garden. There are lots of farm animals that I care for. I milk a goat and I take care of the plants and the garden.

D: How old are you?

S: I'm a young woman in my twenties. My name is Elena.

D: Where do you live?

S: Where it's cold, Poland. I'm a gypsy. I have gypsy lineage, but I have settled on land. I broke away, I got tired of traveling. I wanted to grow things.

D: What are the types of things you grow?

S: Food, herbs. Food for my animals.

D: Go now to the time just prior to your death. Tell me what's going on.

S: It's just dark. There's someone holding me, both arms, from each side. They took me out of my garden, made me go with them.

D: What was their reason for taking you out of your garden?

S: They thought I was someone I wasn't. They thought I was doing something I wasn't.

D: Prior to passing over, what were the lessons you learned in that lifetime?

S: I like the earth, the plants, and the animals. I don't need people. They're too mean.

D: Is that a lesson you learned or is that something you left with?

S: I left with.

D: Then ask your subconscious and Higher Self, is it time to remove that negative thought about people from your subconscious?

S: Yes.

D: Allow yourself to release it from your mind, from your energy. Just because some humans are mean and cruel does not mean they all are. Is it now time to pass over?

S: Yes.

(Now passing over to the other side.)

D: Is there anyone coming to greet you?

S: It has turquoise green eyes. It's a Hathor, very different.

(According to Webster's Dictionary, the meaning of Hathor is: Egyptian Religion, the goddess of love and joy, often represented with the head, horns, or ears of a cow.) In this instance, the client refers to Hathor as "he," yet further on states the Hathor as "male/female" energy.

D: Continue going forward. Tell me what is going on.

S: Hathor is wearing a long robe, very simple, is iridescent and shimmers. He asks me to follow to a place where there's a council.

D: Allow yourself to go to the council. Tell me when you have arrived.

S: Now they're all different.

D: How many are there?

S: I think there's eight.

D: Describe the area.

S: It's just a soft light; there's no furniture. Everyone can just move around, they kind of float around. They can come closer and be more defined and then retreat, sort of into a mist, but you can still see them. They're not sitting; nothing is stagnant. Everything is kind of moving and shifting and changing, always floating around.

D: Where is the Hathor?

S: He stands on my left.

D: As you look at the council, is there a guide or main master?

S: Just the Hathor that came after me, came for me.

D: As you look at each one of the council, allow yourself to describe what each one is wearing.

S: They all look like aliens!

D: Allow each one to come forward, and ask why he is there as your guide.

S: They are from my – where I come from, where I go.

D: Where is that?

S: Pleiades. They're all different. They come from different sections of the Pleiades. Some have very big eyes and very little bodies; others are transparent. Some look a lot like we do with shiny bodies and just the skin. Some of them are wearing robe-like clothing that is kind of see through or shimmering. It's more as if they don't have arms and legs that are defined. Their eyes are so big and deep. Some of them have little bitty hands without real fingers. It's like a baseball mitt, and so they can touch and grasp and pick up things, almost like a suction cup. They're friendly and kind.

D: Ask if one will come forward.

S: The Hathor.

D: Then ask him to come forward. Ask him why he is here for you.

S: He has been connected with me for a long time. He's been keeping track of me, knows everything about me. The others assist.

D: How has he been keeping track of you?

S: There are records.

D: What do you mean by records?

S: It's like a hologram on a tube – a metal tube that is dropped into a light machine and the light produces a hologram. It's like watching a movie. It's like a story that can go forward or backward with the mind or focus. The hologram can move fast or slow. Most of this information was created ahead of time, but only so far into the future. The Council would decide how the hologram – what information it would contain for the next life and what would happen. And then we would go into council again to create the next hologram for the next life. Sometimes more than one life would be created in order to complete – in order to complete with more than one person or event or lesson. But most of the times it was only one, maybe three lives, were programmed at a time. But there was review after each life, even when two or more were created. And they're showing me how that works. It's a copper tube, and the light machines are covered with symbols that represent different events and other souls that were interactive with me in each life. So, great amounts of history can be condensed into those little marks on the copper tube. The other ones continue to shape shift into different forms, constantly changing like shimmering lights, almost like a borealis. If I want to see them, they can take a form and present themselves.

D: Ask if any of them would like to come forward so that you may find out why they are each there for you, for what specific reason. What is it you are to learn from them?

S: They bring the colored lights. They are the colored lights I see. They are the colored lights I see all the time. They show me the lights of a person. They stand behind a person and they show me the light, different colors, so that I may know about that person. They're constantly with me. They're like the fairies that I think I'm seeing. They're like the elementals; they're always around me. They're why I see the light. They just help me know – they help me know I'm not alone. They have fun. They work together; they're always together and they're constantly swirling and changing. But they're the happy energy that I feel all the time. They're like sparkles.

D: The Hathor says he monitors you. Has he instilled any implants within you to help monitor you?

S: No. His eyes are the big eyes I always see. When I close my eyes, those are his eyes. It's not a him, it's male/female. Those are the big eyes, big huge eyes, that are right in front of my face when I close my eyes, so there are no implants.

D: You mentioned different souls that come and go along your journey.

S: The others, the Council, the lights, they're the lights.

D: And other people along your path in different lifetimes. Why were you and I brought together? What is our connection?

S: There is a place being prepared. There are changes that are going to come that will bring a great deal of turmoil for human beings. When the time comes, we are to stand like stanchions, like a pier has many places where the rope can be tied from the boat. We are to be like those stanchions, to call the people who are in turmoil, who are – they're like bouncing around in the choppy water and they need anchors – anchoring. So we will stand like pillars as they move through this room, this space. That will allow them to calm down. It will be through our vibration that calms them. It will be a sound vibration, like a voice and demeanor of not vibrating like they do, changes their vibration. It calms them down. It releases them from their reactionary emotional state into a clear being. They are being prepared for transport. There are activities that we do as we stand like stanchions, like pillars, as they pass through this area. There are others like us that slow them down. It's like a breakwater that you build out into the ocean to protect the harbor. We're like the breakwater that changes the choppy to smooth. Water changes from choppy to smooth – is the emotions of the people. There will be many, many people that will come to the breakwater that we provide. This causes the calming of emotions for transport into the next arena, the next room, the next place, where they will go in transition during this time. It is a purpose that we prepared for long ago. We have known about this time for a long time. We will be able to buffer the way; we are strong. Their energy will be very choppy, but our energy will be fortified in such a way that they do not affect us; we affect them. Our purpose is to help through the changing times, to help as many souls through this gateway.

D: Will this be done on the physical plane?

S: Every dimension you can think of, every dimension that you know, and some that are even more subtle that have not been discovered yet in your human experience. You know about this from the ethereal but not from your perspective; however, you will begin to learn about that as it happens. The vibration will not need to be learned, it's already known, but you will awaken to these other subtle energies as they happen and become aware of them from your human perspective. There will be many that will help in this life. You will need to know; you will interact with many, many people. They will come to you without asking; you don't have to ask. There's nothing for you to do. It will not be like they call for an appointment. It may happen as you're walking down the street or driving your car. You may be interrupted in order to hold energy for someone. If you go to the store, as you walk in the store, your energy will change people who are frantic. You don't have to worry about them hurting you; they can't. Your vibration is your protection. Your vibration, when it becomes refined to do this work, cannot be interrupted, cannot be changed, cannot be altered in any way. That is when you will be completely a channel of energy that will be stronger than anything in its presence.

D: What is the time frame that this will occur for both you and I?

S: These days are coming soon. There will be panic. When there is panic you will know and there is nothing that you can do to increase the vibration now. It will happen automatically. It's built into your DNA as a trigger action to the panic of others to you.

D: Will you and I be working closely together in other areas in the future in this lifetime?

S: Yes. Because we have been selected to stand like stanchions, there will be a need to interact with each other, you and I and many others, which is a way of combining our energy, strengthening our energy, our vibrational field. We will come together like tuning forks to activate each other and we will also need to support each other in knowing, just in knowing that we're not alone, that we're not working alone. Because when the emotional sea begins to move, we will not be in touch with each other. We will be completely surrounded by the emotions of others to transmute and prepare them for transport. But there will be many occasions where we will come together in order to fortify and sustain each other and be support systems for each other, to share wisdom, to share information, to share procedures or standing like stanchions. These comings together will change and vary in a lot of different ways. Sometimes it is just to enjoy life; sometimes it's to share information that is deeply concerning in order to have awareness and knowing before events. Each time it will strengthen all of us as we come together. We know who we are and we will connect very synchronistically, without having to worry about where we are and who is with us, who is another one of us or not. It will become apparent, very clear. Hence, we do this work and move through these fields of energy. There is a place that is prepared for us which is where we will do this work. It is like this room, but it's the – it is not a place, it's not one place, it has a vibrational field. The field itself fortifies us. It will run through our body from top to bottom, bottom to top and from side to side. It will be completely enclosed and enveloped with this field of energy. The field of energy will run through us like the magnetic cycle. People will pass through. It's like the scrubbers at the car wash; we will be like scrubbers. When people pass through, it changes their vibration and helps them drop their fear and panic. We can see the panic in their eyes and feel the choppy vibration from them. But because this place, this field of energy is so strong, they will not affect us.

D: Thank you. Is there any more information for your future that Hathor can bring forth that you will be doing in your current lifetime?

S: Many new experiences will open up, but it will be necessary for me to remember just to enjoy and not to worry about the work, but just to enjoy. Enjoy the sunshine, enjoy the plants, the animals, the people, time to just enjoy and everything will happen naturally. There will be teachings and who wants to learn will be brought to me without putting out invitations or call. They will come to me; they will know when to speak to me or to find me. They will know when they have found me. Sometimes they will come and sit and visit, and maybe we share food, but mostly we sit and talk and when they go away they feel more comfortable. There will be a need to speak more about what I can see. There will be people interested to know that and they will come.

D: And will this vision increase for you?

S: Yes. It will continue to evolve as the needs of the people evolve and change.

D: There was a question you wanted to ask. How your work will change and what will you be doing? Has this been answered, or is there more information to come forth?

S: The writing will begin and it will not be published. It will be through the Internet distribution, in a way published, but not like a book. That work will not remain as information that is like, put down in a book, because this information will change. It cannot stay in a book because the information will not last forever, so it will not be published in the normal way. It will be on the Internet, as the shimmering light that shifts and changes all the time. It will be new, incoming. Preparing other stanchions will be part of the work as well. There will be trips to places where energy needs to be anchored and perhaps other stanchions activated in a very subtle way. It might be missed by everyone involved, but the activation takes place and that's all that's necessary.

D: Is it now time to leave the Council?

S: Yes.

D: Then thank the Council for their help as you leave. Allow yourself now to go to your soul group, and as you go to your soul group, tell me what is going on, in detail.

S: They are the other stanchions; the soul group is the other stanchions. I can see you; I can see many other people. They're all looking at me.

D: As you look at me, what color do you see me projecting to you?

S: Just as you are now in this lifetime, and the color is a baby blue – from the sound of your voice – the sound of your voice and the vibration. There are many others. They are all smiling, an inner knowing.

D: Are there any others that you recognize in your current lifetime?

S: Yes.

D: Would you like to identify the ones that stand out to you?

S: There's so many. Some are surprising. You wouldn't think that they were in this group but they are. So the way they act in this lifetime at this time is not in alignment with who they truly are. Some act very negative, but are here to be stanchions, just not ready yet, have not changed their vibrations. In these cases, when the time comes, the shift will be more impactive to them, and so we will also be using our energy to bring them into alignment when the time comes.

D: Is there anyone else within your soul group that comes forward; that stands out from the others?

S: My daughter.
D: What color is she?
S: Pink.
D: What does that represent to you?
S: Love.
D: Is there anyone else that stands out?
S: Gina.
D: What color does she vibrate?
S: She is green.
D: And what does that represent to you?
S: Her heart that sings.
D: Is there anyone else?
S: Melody. She is white. She will work from the other side. There will be a sandwiching of dimensions as these souls move through this area. There will be those who are in physical body and those that are not, that will sandwich these people as they move through that time period. It is a time continuum, so that it will take a period of time for them to move through and it will also be when their soul is ready in that time.
D: What is the intention of the soul group?
S: To assist, to be midwives, to be spiritual helpers, volunteers like Red Cross, to facilitate the changing of energies. It will be jarring at times, but will dissipate as the vibration shifts, so the more of us working at any one time will reduce the jarring of the energy. Sometimes there will be more people ready to work. Those that have not shifted their energy yet, that are to be stanchions, will have to be called into service. And so in the beginning, the energy will be more jarring until they all are ready to work. When everyone is working together that is supposed to in that space, then the jarring will decrease rapidly as they increase in number. They will not be ready until the shock waves hit them, shifts their energy.

There are others who are ready because they know. Some are still asleep, but will know in the shift.

D: Thank you. Is it time now to leave your soul group and continue forward?

S: Yes.

D: Then give yourself time to say goodbye to them. And now allow yourself to go to the time prior to being born into your next lifetime, where you are able to pick out your physical body. Tell me in detail what is going on.

S: A hologram is showing bits and pieces from other lifetimes are being brought together in a new configuration. One of those components would be a love of the earth, the plants, the trees, the overall matrix of the earth plane, including the water that creates the rainbows that are in the sky and the water, and the moisture that helps the little sparkling light guides to remain active through the water, in different forms like a mist for them. And also there will be trauma added to this body in order to show others. It is like a teaching tool. There will be encounters with certain people for the shifting of old karma. In fact, some of the most accumulated karma will need to be cleared this lifetime in order for this great shift to take place.

D: And has it now, at this point, been cleared?

S: Yes. There were certain structural factors that would keep you in a certain mode; otherwise, a different path would be taken because of the physical body.

D: Have you been on the correct path?

S: Yes. I tried to detour, but was brought back into alignment. A part of me wanted to play and not work. Was not happy about the times that would come and would try to avoid that work, but it cannot be avoided, so everything is in divine order now.

D: And you are in agreement with it now?

S: Yes.

D: And now, before you leave the other side of the veil, is there any more information to be brought forth that will help you, or is there any other place you wish to go to?

S: No.

D: Now that you have much work to do in the future, may I ask Hathor if there will be any more setbacks within the physical body in the future, or is it now in the past?

S: It is in the past.

D: Thank you. Is there any more information before you leave the other side of the veil?

S: Just to say goodbye.

D: As you say goodbye, allow their colored lights, their energy and Hathor's beautiful eyes and energy to fill you with their love, their caring, their guidance, knowing you are never alone. They are always with you. Are you ready to leave now?

S: Yes.

End of session.

During the discussion that followed, Sarnie told me she had always seen colored lights above people's heads and around rooms. She said she now had an understanding that it was her guides, always with her and helping her understand the people she was dealing with. Whenever she would meditate, she would see these huge eyes. In the past she thought it was the eyes of Buddha; now she realizes it is the eyes of a Hathor. She also understands why she was plagued with so many illnesses and operations in her lifetime, and was accepting of her life and what she was here to do.

Sarnie has finished chemotherapy and has been free of cancer for over a year. She said she now believes "the cancer was a trauma to my body in order to show new information to others." She received a letter from an acquaintance that expressed how she had changed their mind about chemo because of the way she handled it.

I have had several clients who have become aware via hypnosis that they were predisposed to a sickness or illness for reasons instilled within the subconscious. For example, during a hypnosis session a client was visited by her reference to a guide, saying she came into her lifetime with a predisposition toward diabetes. She became aware that at the age of two, she was shook violently by her mother which instilled the diabetes within her cellular level, then physical abuse by her husband at the age of twenty-three triggered the diabetes. With its onset as an adult, she said her guide impressed her with the fact that the diabetes was a constant reminder to monitor her food intake and the well-being of her body.

"No soul is forced back into incarnation," according to the book, *Jesus Teacher and Healer,* from White Eagle's Teaching:

> A soul comes back directed by the Higher Self...call it God if you like, but the intuition sends that soul back into incarnation...It may even be that the soul sees that by incarnation in a certain family it will be liable to a certain problem of health, because the tendency towards that disease or disability will be transmitted. The soul will be told: "You can enter into that life, tackle that problem, and see if you can rise above it; it is not necessary for you to suffer if you can bring into operation the law of love."

GLADYS

Four years earlier Gladys went to a hypnotist, after which she began speaking three ancient languages. She stated that at first she didn't know what she was saying and the languages were intermixed, but as time went on the languages began separating within her and an understanding of the words became clear. She believed she was receiving information from a higher level of consciousness. She wanted to find out more about herself.

Gladys has been age regressed and is now in her mother's womb:

D: You are now in your mother's womb, in the embryo stage. How old are you?

G: (Begins speaking in undistinguishable language, which I will refer to throughout her session as UL.) I'm not Gladys.

D: Who are you?

G: I'm Nakalakaha (I spelled this the way it sounded). It was my sacred name. I was given permission by the soul who was to be Gladys to take over her body as a special mission, as she would not have made it to full term. She agreed to leave at this time and thus I took over the body that was made as Gladys, and I made it so she would be carried to full term, and thus she gets to experience through me as a spirit being the life as Gladys that she should have been, but would not have made it.

D: And what is your special mission?

G: To bring light and love and ascension to the world and to those who are upon it at this time.

D: Is there any more information before we leave this time?

G: What do you wish to know?

D: Whatever you wish to bring forth that will help the Gladys that is now in the body.

G: Are you speaking of me, Nakalakaha?

D: Yes.

G: (UL) I see all things. I know all things - past, present, future.

D: Why is this information kept from the consciousness of the body you have inhabited?

G: She has too much fear. I have not truly connected with her fully in this body. There's still Gladys watching over her from the spirit world and sometimes this gets in the way.

D: Can this be removed in time?

G: Yes. She's already working on it. This body known as Gladys is doing well.

D: Thank you. Now allow the physical form, the embryo form, to become younger and younger.

G: Are you talking about Nakalakaha or Gladys?

D: It is your choice.

G: I will return as myself, Nakalakaha, so you may know the true self that is in this body known as Gladys. (UL)

D: Is it time to go to the other side of the veil, or is it necessary to go into the past lifetime known as Gladys?

G: No, you don't need to go into the past life as Gladys, but if you need to know who I truly am, you may go into my past lifetime if you wish.

D: And do we have permission to do so?

G: Yes you do.

D: Then allow yourself to go into your past life and bring forth whatever information you deem necessary.

G: I am her Royal Highness, Serena Ganoctahonach, from Sirius. I love this world. I chose to come here to experience the human form and to help with the ascension process that is now upon the earth. My father was king Oyhashnictahaniachi, (spelled as sounded) great ruler of Sirius. For a time frame, I would say from your time of Christ, 1 A.D., about six million years ago. We lived long lives. We are not mortal as you call it; we are etheric or spiritual beings. We had body shapes. We can create whatever shape we wish. I was female. That was my rank, daughter of the king, Priestess of the highest. That is why I have knowledge of past, present, and future. I work as an emissary of the Creator of all things. I am still on my journey to return to him also. I am just ahead of you a few billion years. I created this form you know as Gladys that I might experience a mortal life as well. And I also had past lives as Isis and Mary of Bethany and many others that I might continue my soul journey as well and experience these things. But I am on a scale different than yours as far as knowledge of the cosmos and spirituality. Gladys' stress that she's experiencing right now is that my separating from – I don't know how to explain it – my soul path as Gladys is putting a little bit of extra strain on Gladys, but she's going through the ascension process and that's part of it. We will continue together as an ascended being. (UL) When she awakens from this hypnosis session, I will have left with her a gift of more knowledge of things to occur, and at this time you may continue to ask your questions to help her in this process. I will be standing by to assist you.

D: Do we now have permission to go to the other side of the veil prior to the form of Gladys being born?

G: Yes, you may do so.

D: Allow yourself now to go to the other side of the veil prior to the incarnation in the form as Gladys.

G: I'm on the other side with Gladys. We're standing together. I was her mother at one time, a long time ago. I am the mother of her form, of her soul.

D: Slowly move forth, and as you become comfortable, find your soul group. Tell me in detail what is happening.

G: Be more specific what you are talking about. Do you want Gladys, the person who left the body at six months, or Nakalakaha? Which one, or both?

D: Which one would be more informative to help the body of Gladys continue her work in her current lifetime?

G: Actually, both.

D: Then allow both to come into view, and you may decide between the two whenever it is necessary.

G: I will speak of Gladys first, as I am mother of her soul. She was birthed from Sirius as well. She will continue. She did not make it through in this mortal life as a soul; she's continuing on her journey as well on this plane. She will reincarnate on planet earth when it recovers from the ascension period and she will continue on her soul journey as well. This physical body is just a vehicle that we both used and now I am using it at this time, and I will continue with its elements as an ascended being. Gladys has chosen to go on a different path. She is still in, as you would call kindergarten; she is a young soul. She's only had thirty or forty birth lives. She wishes to continue her soul journey and she is doing well. She's full of light and love. She is what you would call a gold-ray baby. She was born on Sirius in much advancement of spirituality, so her goals have quickened. She is about – she has many lives on many planets ahead, but I would say she has about five billion lives to go as different souls on different planets and different levels before she returns to the great Creator and becomes one with him again. I will speak more of myself, as I am inhabiting this body as Gladys. I came to earth for the first time as a Lemurian in the early stages of creating the earth. I lived as an etheric spiritual being first during the dinosaur period and watched over the creation of this first civilization. We did not have mortal bodies as you know it, but we were upon the earth and watched over many things. I had a great love for the plant life here, and for the ocean and the seas, and thus we created the first civilization upon the earth and the first beginning of what you eventually would call man, although it was not a man at that time, but just a body of a being starting out on his journey in the mortal form. He did not have the technology or knowledge. He is what you would call Homagnon, or earlier species in the cave-man days, as you would call it. They had intelligence to a certain degree and they lived among the dinosaurs, which is why they find footprints that look humanoid, although they are not human, as you would think of the human in modern times. They lived more off their instinct and survival skills.

My next life was the first mortal form, here you would call it a mortal form, between what you would call my Lemurian or etheric form or my first actual mortal physical form, 450,000 BC. We were of a slower vibrational rate, so we appeared physical but we weren't quite mortal. I was still considered Lemurian, but it was more a true Lemurian by then. We had descended and walked upon the earth in highly spiritual, more physical forms. We were priests and priestesses. We were organizing the spiritual realm upon the earth, creating a spiritual hierarchy that would watch over the earth, creating the akashic records on the spiritual, etheric level, and thus we did walk upon the earth for many hundreds of thousands of years.

D: May I ask a question at this time?

G: You may.

D: What is our connection, my ancient self and you during that time? Because we are brought together now, I feel we have connections from the past.

G: You were Archangel Ariel when the world was first conceived when I was still living upon Sirius. We knew of you. We had spoken to each other on a spiritual level. You were a higher spiritual being of light than I was at that time. You were sent by the Creator of all things to oversee the spiritual gifts and blessings from him. You brought those forth from a different dimension or different area of the cosmos. You brought that forward into the void with him. You brought those things to the earth to help create the spiritual womb as the world would be formed in, and that is one of our connections. You were birthed onto Lemuria as well and came down to a more spiritual solid form as I was in Lemuria, although you worked in a different location, more toward China; I was more toward Tibet. We had knowledge of each other and spiritual connections then as well through higher sources, although we never personally met upon the earth in physical, semi-physical bodies. We are connected through the cosmos and that's our connection at that time in Lemuria. We have been (UL) I'm thinking of our soul groups. You're like an older sister in a spiritual sense of a soul group. Your soul group as Ariel was of an earlier birthing from our Father, the Creator, where as I was younger. Our soul groups are connected in the sense that your soul group is like an older sister to my soul group, and that's our very first connection. So you understand, our soul groups travel together throughout our many lifetimes in the different forms in our journeys as our souls. So we are connected throughout the entire journey of our souls.

D: How many are on your Council?

G: There are five.

D: Will each come forward individually so that she may know why each one is there specifically for her, and what knowledge she is to gain from them?

G: (UL) Fubbi Quantz is here. He is my ancient Avatar teacher from China – Tibet. It was from him that I learned about mathematics and geometry. He reminds me of all the things that I know of the cosmos, and he is a spiritual guide for those things to be brought back into my memory at this time and in the future. He is stepping back. And Shemesh, my Egyptian guide is here. He has knowledge of the resurrection and the ascension process as well as Egypt, the pyramids of Giza, the machines and the knowledge I had back then. Michael, the Guardian Angel is here. He is here to help me remember the things I have brought with me as Nahalakala. My next guide, (UL) my other guide is my father, as Gladys' father Joe, just to bring me love and light and comfort when I need it. The other guide that is there is a mother, a female presence. (UL) She does not wish to give her sacred name at this time. But know that she will, and is here as a female guide for the female energy that is in me. She is from Sirius, of the higher order of the priesthood that is there.

D: Take a look at their robes and tell me the color.

G: They are white and iridescent and gold and purple, depending on which one you are looking at.

D: Look at each one, breaking it down for the knowledge it brings forth.

G: Fubbi Quantz is wearing pure white and iridescent. It represents healing and a great white light of an Avatar, also connected with the great white light of the Father, Creator of all things.

D: Is there anything hanging around his neck?

G: There is a crystal.

D: Look at the crystal and bring forth the information from it.

G: (UL) Permission is granted. All the knowledge of the crystal has now been put into my mind, to my spirit and my soul that I shall remember it when I need it.

D: Move on to the next one.

G: Shemesh is wearing white and gold, glittering gold that represents purity and knowledge, truth in its most purest form. Michael is wearing pure white light of the Father. He is surrounded by the pure white light and because it is pure, it radiates all colors of the rainbow that represents the love of the Father in its purest form. My father is wearing purple for royalty, for he is a descendant of Jesus Christ, and that is of the line of David, and thus my bloodline runs. It represents the bloodline of the Holy Grail. (UL) I am not to describe what my mother is wearing. It is too sacred at this time. (UL) They say I have all that I need. They will continue to be with me and guide me as I need it, but my third eye has been awakened fully that I may receive all that I need from this time forth.

D: Go to the time just prior to being born into your current lifetime. Why was the physical form known as Gladys picked?

G: Because of her bloodline and because she was of me as well, and because of her mother. The DNA that her mother had is the pure bloodline. It was needed as it had the knowledge still in it that was required for Nakalakaha to return to perform these things. So it was chosen.

D: Were there other physical forms for the choosing?

G: No. This was the only form available at this time that was needed. That is why the form who was to be Gladys stepped out.

D: Go now to the school of learning and describe what you see.

G: Are you talking about the Akashic Record Library?

(Akashic Records is defined as: "That out of which all things are formed; tiny, ethereal records that store attitudes, emotions, and concepts from the mental mind as the physical body experiences tastes, smells, sights, sounds, emotions, and thoughts during each earthly incarnation.")

D: Yes.

G: Do you wish to see the outside of the building first?

D: Allow it to come forth as you wish.

G: It is made of gray marble, beautiful swirling marble of white and gray, pure and translucent, specks of gold of the highest spiritual quality, and thus spiritual knowledge is right within the walls. It is about what you would call ten stories high. It has beautiful angles like crystals do on the outer walls. The doors are pure gold, not like the gold you think that is shiny. It is translucent. So pure a gold that it is translucent and you can walk right through it, and as you enter you are purified. The hallways are full of the great, white light of the Creator. You go by thought to where you need to. It shows you everything that you ask for and all that you stand in need of at that time, and you will be directed to where you need to go within the library. It is actually on the inside formless, and yet has form as you need it. You create it as you need it with your thoughts. There are many different levels and dimensions within this building that you can enter. It is like, if you need to learn about the stars, you would enter that door and go into a separate room that is like the stars at night, a planetarium. You would learn of the cosmos and different things, yet it can transport you from that room directly to a planet or to a different area or dimension. You feel like you are sitting there, but can transport yourself and learn about that place and experience it for yourself and then come back. Then if you wish to learn about animals or creatures or snakes or whatever you wish, you could be taken to that. If you wish to read a book on that, you would be taken to a book, or if you wish to be taken to a planet to see how that creature lives, you could experience it like that. So it is multidimensional. It is almost what you would call on Star Trek, the hologram room. Sort of like that but different.

D: Why were Gladys and I connected in this lifetime?

G: Because it was your destiny. You made prior agreements before coming into these lives to meet. You had a great love for each other and you knew each other in many lives. You actually got to meet each other as soul groups. It was part of your destiny to come here and to fulfill these things. Your heart was full of love and compassion for Gladys, as she was struggling in this life as Gladys. You will have many lives together yet in the future, as well in assisting one another in your souls' journey.

D: Are there any other questions that Gladys has before leaving?

G: No. All has been answered.

End of session.

Gladys is now calm and at peace within herself. She believes there is a higher purpose for her life here on earth and is presently studying with a shaman.

Chapter 8

Transformation

This chapter is devoted entirely to a woman who was so stressed she could barely talk over the telephone without crying. Her life appeared to be at the bottom of a dark well, but through hypnosis she was able to climb up from that well and free her emotional binds. She made great strides in her life in a short period of time. The changes occurred in three hypnosis sessions, several hours each session. Generally each session is one week apart, but since she had a busy schedule and became a client just prior to the holidays, they were spread over a period of six weeks. This is not to say everyone will be able to reach such emotional freedom within three sessions as each person is working on their own issues, but it shows how "unveiling the past can heal the future."

MADGE

My first meeting with Madge was at a workshop we were attending. Each individual was asked to briefly tell a little about himself or herself. During break, Madge introduced herself, saying she had been searching for someone in my field. After a few moments of discussion, I gave her my card. Two months later, Madge called, breaking down almost immediately. She could barely get the words out, so we set up an appointment

SESSION 1

When she walked into my office, her physical appearance was almost masculine. She was a single woman in her early fifties, of stocky build, with her hair pulled back in a bun and very little, if any, makeup. Her long pants and shirt made me think of someone who was hiding behind her clothes. As she spoke, her voice began quivering. She said, "I don't know which way to turn. I feel all used up." She was beginning to have panic attacks. Over the past ten years, she had put on thirty extra pounds. She said, "Why is it so hard to accept joy in my life?"

She had never been hypnotized, but appeared eager. After putting her into a deep hypnotic state, we began. (I wish to note, except for name and location changes, the following is being transcribed exactly as it was taken off the tape recording. This is done to keep the integrity of the hypnosis session as Madge removes negative energies, allowing the changes to take place within.)

D: Where are you?

M: I'm at a farmhouse. Mother brings me down here to stay every summer.

D: Where is this farmhouse located?

M: It's in Alabama. I'm a little girl.

D: How old are you?

M: Under six years old.

D: Look around. Is there anyone else there?

M: Tom.

D: Who is Tom?

D: He's my uncle. He's always touching me and messing with me and pinching me. He's just touching me inappropriately.

D: Is there anyone else around?

M: Aunt Anna, but he's mean to her, too.

D: Ask him why is he touching you?

M: 'Cause he's a pervert. Women are just objects.

D: Has he done this before?

M: Yes.

D: Go back to the first time he touched you, when you were younger. Tell me what is going on.

M: Every time mother took me down there, he did that.

D: How old were you the first time?

M: About four.

D: Go to a significant scene. Where are you now?

M: Sitting on his lap. When I was little he would always have me sit on his lap. He would rub himself up against my bottom.

D: Turn around, look him square in his eyes with fire in your eyes, and tell him to stop!

M: (Loudly speaking.) Stop it! Don't touch me anymore! Don't touch me! I want to get down.

D: What he did was wrong. Tell him.

M: What you did was wrong! Don't touch me. I'm going to the kitchen to be with Aunt Anna.

D: Before you go into the kitchen, turn around. What would you like to do to him?

M: (Loud voice.) I would like to smack him right in the shins!

D: Go ahead. Smack him in the shins.

M: He doesn't like it, but I just kicked the hell out of him.

D: Do it again.

M: (Pause.) Yeah, I kicked him in the other knee, too.

D: Is there anything else you would like to do?

M: No, because his legs hurt him already.

D: Tell him, you are a small child. He is taking advantage of you as a small child.

M: I wanted you to love me and take care of me, and you abused me. I want you to leave me alone. I don't love you anymore. (Voice rising again.) Don't touch me ever again!

D: Tell him, what he has done to you is his problem; it is not your problem. He is wrong.

M: You're wrong in doing this. You've hurt me. I'm just a child. I'm just a baby, and you've done this.

D: You trusted him and he betrayed your trust.

M: Yes, yes he did. You were my family. You were supposed to take care of me and watch over me and you didn't. I don't ever want you to touch me again. I don't ever want you to touch me again, ever!

D: Scan your body. The pain you feel, has it created physical pain in your body?

M: I have herpes on my genital.

D: Go to that area. Ask your Higher Self, is it time for you to remove this pain that you've been holding onto?

M: Yes, it is. It's time for it to be healed.

D: Then completely encircle it with a color. And what would this color represent?

M: Aqua water, cool water.

D: Encircle the entire area with the color aqua. And now, with your imaginary water, flush it out completely, allowing the water to drain down your body and out your toes.

D: What color would you like to replace this with? What would it represent to you?

M: Pink. Just good health, good blood flow, just love.

D: You no longer need to hold onto that pain from your uncle. You trusted him and he betrayed that trust. He made you feel unsafe and uncomfortable. That was his problem, not yours. It is time to feel good about yourself.

M: I see myself now with a little dress on. It's made out of flour sack material. I have curly hair.

D: Is there anyone with you?

M: Just Aunt Anna and myself. She said to be careful; there are snakes. But she knows somehow that my life is going to be hard. She was born with a veil over her face. She has second sight. She says I do, too.

D: What else is she telling you?

M: That she knows that Uncle Tom does what he does, but he's a painful man. He hurts her, too. She'll stay with him her whole life. She's trying to prepare me for the pain of being a woman.

D: What is she saying to you?

M: That, just stay close to her; stay close to her.

D: What does she mean by the pain of being a woman?

M: That pain from childbirth. She has problems with menstrual cycles. Whenever she bleeds, she always goes to the outhouse; there's no indoor plumbing. So she's always taking rags to the outhouse. I asked her why she has the rags. She tells me it's because she bleeds. It's the pain of being a woman.

D: How does that make you feel?

M: I don't want to be a woman. I don't want to have any children. I don't want to be in any more pain.

D: Ask her, is it because of her pain that she was going through that she instilled this mental pain in you about being a feminine woman?

M: She was like a child emotionally. (Long pause.) She had a really wonderful trunk in her hallway that she let me look at once. They were treasures in there to me; old hats and feathers and eggs that didn't have anything in them.

D: There is joy and wonderful experiences in being a woman. Call in your Higher Self. Ask, is it time to remove these negative thoughts about being a woman, about being feminine, about being a female, about the things she said to you which were not accurate?

M: (Deep sigh.) Yes, it's time.

D: Ask your Higher Self to help guide you to remove those inner thoughts.

M: Yes, she confused me. Higher Self, please help me. He's touching my face. (Deep sigh.) It's like a father would reach down and put his hand underneath his child's chin, turns the face up so they can look at him, so that they'll know that they're loved.

D: Do you now feel that love deep within?

M: Yes.

D: Allow that love to grow within you.

M: (Loud crying.) I just wanted to be loved! (Continual sobbing.)

D: Just allow those negative thoughts from your childhood to be released. All those negative thoughts you've held onto all your lifetime, allow them to flow out and be released. Remove all those thoughts about not wanting to be feminine; feel it draining out your body. Your Aunt Anna meant well, but she was inaccurate because of the pain and suffering she was going through.

M: It's going on the ground. The earth is soaking it up. It's almost like I'm standing there peeing my pants. It's like I can't believe I'm doing it, I'm just standing there peeing my pants.

D: Just allow it to continue draining from your body.

M: I'm giggling and running around in a circle. I'm playing. It feels good.

D: Allow that feeling to grow stronger within you.

M: I'm playing with the flowers.

D: Smell the flowers. Allow the child within you to play and become stronger. (Pause.) Now allow the child's face to come to you. See the child within you. See the beauty within yourself. Absorb that beauty. Allow that child to become one with you again, to become one with you. Love that child that is you. Hold and nurture that child, that child that is part of yourself.

M: I'm sitting on the front porch at Aunt Anna's and Uncle Tom's place in the rocking chair. I'm just being held on my lap. My face is being held against my chest. I'm humming a tune; my eyes are closed. My baby arms are hugging me now, and I'm just very, very peaceful. I'm resting like a child rests after they've played hard and hurt, and cried themselves to sleep. I have dimples. They show when I smile. I have these special little hands.

D: Why are they special?

M: They sense things when they touch things, the left one especially. Even as a child, even then, I liked to touch the skin of people. It was like I could sense things that were going on with them when I touched them. I guess I always felt it was my fault. Uncle Tom did those things to me because I liked to touch things when I was a child. I like to touch my grandmother's skin on her arms and her face. I like touching my Aunt Anna's arms and hands. Even today, I like touching people on the arm. I like touching their hands especially. I hold their hands and massage them of sorts. It gives me a sense of knowing who they are.

D: Ask your Higher Self, do you have healing powers in your hands?

M: (Pause.) Yes.

D: Think of yourself as a flower, in the bud stage, and now the bud is opening, blossoming, fully opened.

M: (Takes a deep breath, and releases it.) Yes, I'm painting my toenails.

D: Allow that child now to go within you and become one with you again. Allow her to become part of you again.

M: Yes. I feel I'm pregnant. And the baby is inside my stomach now. She's being absorbed in my bones, sweet child, a sweet tiny voice. She's making me laugh. Now she's stopped. I can hear her voice. I can hear her talk to me. It's okay; it's okay. She has such a pretty face, with her own baby eyes. It's okay. She likes running her finger around my mouth.

D: She is the child within. She is you. Is there anything you would like to say to the child, to the true you?

M: I am going to protect you. I am not going to give so much that you leave again. You and I are the same person. We are going to have love and joy in our lives, and you will experience more as a total human being, I promise.

D: Allow the inner child to grow within you; she is you. And now, continue from this day forward to nurture yourself, your inner child.

M: I don't have to give everything to everybody. I have to have some love for me. I have to have some love for me.

D: Now, scan your childhood. Ask your Higher Self, is there a significant event that your Higher Self would like you to go to that you need to deal with, or is it just time to remove the pain and suffering that you have experienced as a child, to finally remove it totally and completely?

M: Yes. (Pause.) Oh, it's bad. We don't have to go there. The baby's safe; the baby's safe.

D: Then allow your Higher Self to remove all pain and suffering from your childhood.

M: It's sweeping it out the door.

D: Discard it. Remove it.

M: It's like the room is barren. It's an old room, but it's barren. She's sweeping it, sweeping it all out the door, down the steps. It's gone.

D: Is there anything else you need to do?

M: Yeah. We need to let some sunshine in.

D: Then let the sunshine in; let it begin pouring in.

M: Just cover it in white light. Cover the whole thing in white light. She's just turning around in a circle, like you were taking a shower. She's making sure that she's covered in it. She's stretching her arms out, rubbing it on herself like it's soap.

D: Would you like to decorate the room now?

M: Yes, oh yes! (Long pause.) It's sturdy, beautiful hardwood floors. The windows are big, so she can look out and see what's going on. There's a corner that's kind of lonely, like she's looking, expecting someone to be there, but there's not anybody there.

D: It's your house, decorate your house, decorate yourself. Take it one step at a time. You have love and joy within yourself.

M: The curtains are sheer, and just kind of drape real easy. They're beautiful, but they just hang there.

D: Would you like to change them?

M: I'd like to have them so that I can pull them closed if I want to, or just tie them back to look at the sunset or sunrise.

D: This is you; this is your house. Decorate it the way you want it to be. Fix those curtains.

M: The windows open, you know. They open and the breeze comes through. She doesn't have to worry about falling out. Now it's not stuffy. In the bed where she was so frightened, in the corner, it's different now. It's soft and warm and beautiful. There's paintings, beautiful paintings.

D: Sense the paintings. Go up to the paintings and look at them.

M: There's a woman in one of them that's sitting in front of a dressing table brushing her hair. Looks just like me.

D: Is this you?

M: Yes. There's a chair sitting by a small table. She sits at it. She likes to read; she likes to wonder about the questions coming to her mind.

D: Allow yourself to nurture yourself.

M: She's making tea. It's an old fashioned kitchen. She wants it to be bigger, but she likes the big window in the kitchen, too. It's a different window from that other window. The kitchen is different. It's warm. She makes little things to go with the tea. She's smiling sweetly because she has two cups and two saucers out. She's expecting someone to come over that she loves so dearly.

D: You refer to she. Who is she?

M: She is me.

D: Then talk about yourself. She is you. She is not another person.

M: She's wondered if it wasn't somebody else inside.

D: No, it is you. Incorporate her within yourself. Allow her to become part of you.

M: She gave up her beauty because other people didn't want her to have it. She gave it away.

D: And what does she want?

M: She's opening her door. (Gasps.) She just threw her arms around my neck! I'd love to stay. Outside and inside look different. Outside's gray and cold; inside is a warm place. (Pause.) Oh, it's so funny. It's like I'm being a young woman, like being thirty. I'm altogether now; I'm two people in one.

D: But together, this is you. Ask your Higher Self.

M: Oh, yes, this is me.

D: Then ask your Higher Self to bring them together. Bring the different parts of yourself together to become one. It is time. Ask your Higher Self.

M: Yes, it's time.

D: Then bring the different parts of you together. You have brought the child within yourself. Now (she cuts me off.)

M: The dressing table in the painting is sitting in the room now. She's just sat there and looked at herself in the mirror and realized that she's the same.

D: Allow her to become part of you, a beautiful woman.

M: She's looking at her hands again, something about her hands.

D: Take a look at her hands. What do you see?

M: It's like, she has this passion in her hands. When she touches a person, its – she embraces love. Children, animals, plants, people. (Begins to cry.)

D: Tell me what's going on.

M: She's an Indian woman. She was thrown off a cliff.

D: Why was she thrown off a cliff?

M: Because she had second sight, she was thrown off a cliff.

D: Go into the second sight.

M: She knew about the seasons; she knew about the plants; she knew about all the things. The white men threw her off a cliff; they destroyed them all. They beat her; they beat her.

D: Go into that fear you are holding onto.

M: I'm lost. I don't know how to get back to the woman sitting at the table.

D: Don't worry about it. Stay with the Indian woman at this time. Go into the fear in the Indian woman about having second sight.

M: (Starts crying loudly.) They killed her! They killed him – her mate. I want her! They threw them both off the cliff.

D: If you wish to look at this as a movie or continue to go through it, allow yourself to do so. It is your choice.

M: (Crying lessens, then stops.)

D: Now, go into that second sight, to the pain that she has received from losing her mate, from being beaten, then thrown off a cliff. Where is she holding onto that pain of having second sight?

M: They raped her. She cannot have – she can't – she is promised.

D: What is she promised? What are you promised? This is you we are talking about. What are you promised?

M: They are soul mates; they are soul mates.

D: Look at him. Take a look at him.

M: He's a fine man.

D: Do you recognize him as someone in your current lifetime?

M: I don't know if he's the same person or not. I think it's wishful thinking.

D: Just allow it to come forward. You can analyze it later.

M: He's an Ohio plumber. Yes, I do.

D: Go back to the pain you are holding onto for having second sight. Where in your body are you holding onto the pain? Scan your body.

M: Just on the sides of my eyes, on my temple.

D: Go into the eyes on the sides, the temples, the pain you have received for having second sight. This is a gift, a wonderful, beautiful gift that people killed you because of. Ask your Higher Self; is it time to remove this pain?

M: Yes.

D: Then completely encircle the pain on the sides of your eyes and your temples. If you were to give it a color, what color would it be?

M: It's yellow. It's like a crown. It's made out of glass, kind of. It looks like it would go on a big statue or something, from years ago. It's been there for centuries.

D: Ask yourself, is this part of the pain that needs to be removed?

M: No, she asked to wear it. It's part of her. She's had it forever.

D: Keep your crown on, but remove the pain.

M: People don't like it.

D: Remove the pain. Your Higher Self has said it is time to remove the pain and suffering you have received.

M: Yes. (Pause.) It's funny. She just – he loves her so. He loved her before. He's a shaman, to the Indian thing. (Pause.) I saw him before in the Roman times. He looks funny in a toga. She just loves him. She sees him. When she looks in his chest, she sees his light. She was a frail thing.

D: Allow yourself to remove the pain from your temples.

M: She brought babies; you know that, don't you? That's why she doesn't like to do it now. She couldn't stand the children dying anymore. She knew things all the time. She could sense the animals in the forest. She knew where to find things.

She's sacred, white, and they didn't like her. They didn't trust her. She was screaming, begging and screaming. She just left. She just went from one place to the other, like she could transport herself. They're turning around and looking at her, like they don't know what's happened. She walked away from them. The crown's on her head. I can see it. Looks kind of pretty because she's dressed in buckskins. She's looking at her hands again. She's just turning them over and looking at them.

D: Why is she looking at them?

M: Because she realizes they're tools.

D: Have you brought those tools into your current lifetime to use again?

M: Oh, she does, but no one thinks it. She can take her fingers and rub it on the third eye of a crying child and the child will stop crying. When she talks to children, they either see her, or they're totally frightened of her. The ones that see her see a light around her. Sometimes it's like a minute, when other people see it, too. And then she gets tired because people use her energy up. She doesn't know how to – she looks at her hands as tools, with compassion and love, creativity. She has expressiveness in herself. She is passionate.

D: What is her name?

M: Me. It is me.

D: What year is it?

M: It's a timeline that just kind of runs. She wants a new name. She wants somebody to call her by a special name.

D: What is that special name?

M: It's silly; it's honey. She wants someone to call her honey.

D: What year is it?

M: Oh, it's – I don't know. I see the hands.

D: And now, go into your head. Go into your temples. Go into the pain that was put there because of the second sight. Allow your Higher Self to help you to remove the pain. Just take the pain and sweep it out. Are you doing so?

M: Yes.

D: Rinse it out now with cool, clear water. Is it cleaned out now?

M: Yeah. It's cool. It's a sweet herb; it kind of smells like sandalwood. I can see her mixing it up.

D: Then allow her to put it on your temples and your eyes.

M: Yeah.

D: Is she doing so?

M: Yes.

D: You have been given a special gift. You should not have received pain for this gift. That was instilled by people who were not knowledgeable; they were ignorant. You have removed the pain of other peoples' ignorance. That is their problem, not yours. You have been given this special gift. Cherish this gift. If your Higher Self wishes to bring this special gift forward into your current lifetime, allow that to be so.

D: Yes. That's where the berries were. She thought it was something that everybody had. He made her feel that way. He asked her where the deer would be, and she would look over her shoulder and smile, and just tell him like she should already know.

D: Scan that lifetime.

M: She didn't have any children.

D: What were the lessons you learned from that lifetime?

M: That she had the love. He wasn't the most handsome of the men in the tribe, but he loved her. She would not leave him. She would not run away. She could have saved herself, but she stayed. That's why they threw her off the cliff, because she was there, she didn't run away.

D: What did she learn from that?

M: That her love is stronger than anything; that her love is stronger than anything. Oh! Oh, okay, it makes sense. It's the hands, the grasping of the hands. She was ripped apart. She was holding onto him, to the very last minute. That's why she keeps turning her hands over, like they failed her. That's why I keep turning my hands over, looking at them. That was me! (Begins sobbing.) They took him from me.

D: If you wish to view this as a movie, allow yourself to do so, it is your choice.

M: (Crying lessens, then stops.) That's why she was so attuned to the Native American way. It seems so natural; it's part of her spirit, her grandfather. He's an amazing person.

D: It's time now to begin leaving that lifetime, taking yourself higher and higher, look up and see yourself going toward the light. Do you see yourself going toward the light?

M: Yes.

D: Allow yourself to go into the light, taking with you all the joy and happiness, cleansing yourself from all negativity from that lifetime.

M: (Giggles, then deep sigh.)

(Before bringing her out of hypnosis, Madge is taken to a peaceful place to rest and re-energize.)

End of session.

~ ~ ~

Discussion after the session revealed that Madge did not remember much of the negativity from her childhood. She had been continually molested as a small child. As a protective device, she created a separation of her innocent, inner child from the adult she became. That was indicated by the continual reference to herself in the third person, "she." This is why I had Madge integrate the inner child within herself again.

Her Aunt Anna, even though she loved the little girl, was herself not happy with being a woman and so instilled this within Madge. She appeared tired after the session, which can happen after the releasing of much negative energy. She also said she felt "lighter," which many times is the sensation, again with the removal of negative energy. Madge set up an appointment for the following week.

In Dr. Francesca Rossetti's book, *Psycho Regression, A New System for Healing & Personal Growth*, she states:

> The present-day personality is comprised of many likes and dislikes, pet hates and fears, ideas and fixations that have been accumulated over the centuries. Parental emotions and ideologies also help to shape the outer mask of a developing child, but the problems really start to surface when a person continues to look through his or her parents' eyes as an adult, or becomes emotionally frozen because of an unresolved experience when he or she was still a child.

Session 2

The following week when Madge walked into my office, she was cheerful and bubbly. She had her hair cut and styled and was wearing lipstick. She said, "The day after her session, it was as though a funnel had opened up and latent memories began pouring out." She stayed in bed most of the day, crying and sobbing. Madge said she came as close as picking up the telephone to cancel our next appointment, but decided to "stick it out." By the third day, it was like a "new lease on life."

She began looking for another apartment, as "she hasn't been happy with where she was living for years."The session had "freed her to make decisions which before were confusing." In this session, she wants to work on happiness. She wants to find out why she's not letting happiness come into her life. "Let's get started and see where it takes me!" she said.

And the hypnosis begins:

D: Go back to the time of not allowing happiness to come into your life. Look around. Allow it to come into focus. Tell me what you see.

M: I don't see anything.

D: Ask your Higher Self, what is holding you back? Allow it to come into focus.

M: (Long pause.) I'm drowning. I feel like I'm drowning.

D: Tell me what is happening.

M: Just reaching up. All I see is just one hand hanging onto something, the side of a boat or something. The other hand is reaching up toward the sky, and I just feel like I'm drowning. (Long pause.) A man's carrying me, and I'm a small child. I've fallen through the ice and I've drowned.

D: Go back, just prior to the drowning. Tell me what is happening.

M: My brother did it.

D: What did your brother do?

M: He attacked me, tormented me. He was pulling pranks.

D: Do you recognize him as someone in your current lifetime?

M: Oh, yes! He's my brother in this lifetime, my brother Joey.

D: How much older was he when you were in that lifetime?

M: Not very much, maybe three years. It's kind of out in the country. I was very young, maybe six or seven.

D: Why did you go into that lifetime to live only a short period of time? What was to be gained?

M: I was three. Music lessons, girly things. I was a girl, sheltered. I had a special tutor. (Pause.) He hated me; still in that lifetime he hated me. He was cruel in many lifetimes.

D: When you came into that lifetime was it a knowing that your life would be cut short or was it an accident?

M: It was a choice that he made.

D: Was this also a choice that you made?

M: Yes. I had given him an opportunity to pay back karmic debt.

D: What was that karmic debt for?

M: He had been cruel to me in previous lifetimes.

D: How would he have been able to pay back karmic debt?

M: He could have been a big brother, sheltered me, part of a nurturing family, but he chose to torment me once again. He didn't mean for me to die.

D: What were the lessons you learned in that lifetime?

M: Fate has a hand in our lives.

D: What did you learn in that lifetime that will help you in your current lifetime?

M: She's been protected in this lifetime through spirit, a life when she met a man many lifetimes ago. She chose a very hard lifetime. She wants it to be over with. She does not wish to come back.

D: Which lifetime are you referring to?

M: This one.

D: Expand on that.

M: The one that she's in now.

D: Bring forth information from spirit that will help you in your current lifetime.

M: (Long pause.) She has to be more focused. She has to clean up her act. Not everyone, even though they may seem loving, can do what's best for her. They're incapable of it. She's not open. She's shutting light; she's shutting light.

She didn't ask for money; she asked for love. She didn't ask for money; she asked for love. She cannot have one without the other. She has to have relationship. She has to have people in her life. She has to give up the fear. She has to be willing to sacrifice herself in a different way.

D: In what way?

M: She has to let somebody – she has to look at a person's eyes and tell them that she loves them. She has to be willing to have a mate. She sacrificed herself to others, but she couldn't give herself to the right person because her soul mate wasn't in her life. She gave them what she thought they wanted so that they would go away and let her do without. She felt if she paid her debt, she actually could leave. She's trying to get her karma paid so she can leave. She cannot have one without the other.

D: What does she need to do in order to accept the success in her life now?

M: (Long pause.)

D: Tell me what's going on.

M: She's just – she's at the base of a mountain, things falling off of it. Boulders, big rocks falling on her head.

D: What are these boulders representations of?

M: She trusts the wrong people. The gun's being taken out of the cabinet. It's a man's hand; it's a long rifle. It's like, having to protect the house or something, an old place.

D: Look into the man's eyes. Do you recognize him as someone in your current lifetime?

M: My grandfather.

D: Look around. Do you see yourself anywhere?

M: No.

D: Go into another room. Do you see yourself anywhere else?

M: No.

D: Then go up to your grandfather. Ask your Higher Self, what is the significance of him protecting the cabin with a rifle?

M: He's French, French Canadian.

D: What is the importance of this in your current lifetime?

M: I keep running away.

D: What are you running away from?

M: Pain.

D: Where is the pain coming from?

M: Pain, coming from loving. I didn't want the pain of loving.

D: Where are you holding onto this pain of loving?

M: My shoulders.

D: Ask your subconscious; is it time to remove this pain from your shoulders?

M: She's dancing around like a fool! Yes.

D: The pain of loving someone. By removing this pain, will it allow you to begin opening up your heart, accepting someone to love again?

M: Yes, it will.

D: Go into your shoulders. What color would you give the pain?

M: Bright orange.

(I have her remove the pain, spitting it out of her mouth.)

M: Yes, she's spitting. She left that cabin. She's running from the cabin. They were totally different people than what her people are.

(In filling the area where the pain was removed, she decided to fill it with a soft periwinkle color representing love.)

D: And now, you said she ran out of the cabin. Why did she run out?

M: She – running from her family, but they became her family because she wanted to be free. She wanted to go toward the mountain; she wanted to explore. There's a lot of countryside. I recognized it.

D: Was it the right choice?

M: They accepted her, but they – they didn't – they didn't expect her to have her own (choice.) They expected her just to be part of the group. She never had enough. (Long, long pause.) Seeds trying to grow. Seeds trying to grow.

D: What does that mean to you?

M: I don't know. All I see is a rose bush, cut, that's been cut all the way down to the root. No flowers, just thorns.

D: Go into the rose bush.

M: It's not growing in grass, it's growing in mud.

D: Ask your Higher Self, what does that rose bush represent to you?

M: To her, the base is strong. People tried to tear it before; it didn't work. It started growing. It's going to have so many blooms on it that people won't be able to – they're going to take some of the blooms off of it. It won't matter. The blooms will just come back.

D: Ask your Higher Self, is this rose bush representing you?

M: Yes, it is! People are trying to destroy her. But her roots are deep.

D: How can you nurture your rose bush?

M: She has to till the soil, more aeration.

D: What does that mean to you?

M: That I have to take care of myself. I have to be concerned with survival of my roots because I can't bloom if I allow them to rip me out of the soil. Then I bloom. It will be okay if they share in my success, because once I bloom, there will be enough, there will be enough light, sunshine. Beautiful, beautiful.

D: Go into the success of the blooms. What is holding you back from succeeding?

M: She's frightened. She's fearful.

D: Go into the frightened, the fearful.

M: She wants to be her own person! She doesn't want to be what other people want her to be. She wants to be her own person. She wants to be loved for who she is.

D: What is holding you back from being your own person? Go to the cause.

M: She's rubbing the rim of a bowl and singing. I don't see her face; I just see the sleeve on her, kind of like a dressing gown, like a robe. She's praying, tuning this bowl, going through the ritual, but there's no passion in it. She's going through the motions of it. She's peaceful, but there's no passion. There has to be passion in her life. She's shut all the passion out, because she – she didn't want to be used anymore. She has to get back to passion. She's trusting, but (long pause.)

D: Tell me what's going on.

M: There's a war going on. One soldier is smiling at another soldier. Two men. They're not in this lifetime. It's just as though they're getting ready to drop a bomb, but the plane's on the ground; it's not off the ground; it's on the ground. They're in someplace hot, because their sleeves are rolled up. They're squatted down. They're not American soldiers. English, I think, Australian. They're looking at somebody. They know what's going on. They're in the middle of this conflict, and they're not afraid. No fear. She cannot have fear! She lives her life in fear! Without passion! She cannot have joy without passion. She cannot have passion with fear.

D: Where are you holding onto the fear in your body?

M: Knee, her knee.

D: Go into your knee. Ask your Higher Self, is it time to remove the fear from your knee that keeps you from having passion in your life?

M: Yes. Yes it is.

(She encircles her knee with a color of steel blue and washed it down her legs and out the toes.)

M: Splinters, long, long splinters. Sharp ones.

D: Push them all the way out. (Knee was cleansed with cool, healing water.)

M: She pulverized it. She put it on the base of her rose bush. She has roses at the base, and growth, and I just keep reaching as the rose bush gets older. Roses just keep coming on bigger and bigger. Her knee is filled will strong muscles. These muscles are yellow, strong.

D: And now, you keep referring to she. She is you. She is you. Incorporate her within yourself. She is part of you; incorporate her within yourself. Allow her to become part of you, the beautiful part of you, the passion, the love, the success in life, allow her to become part of you. Incorporate her into you. Are you doing so?

M: Yes. She has to – she has to look and listen to what is being said to her and about her so that she can respond from a non-fearful place. She is (long pause) she's going to be okay. She's climbing a tree. She likes the womanness, so she's not afraid of being a woman, she will do well. She has to have passion in her life.

D: Allow passion to come into your life now. Allow yourself to open up to receive passion and give passion.

(She went to a peaceful place so she could rest before coming out of the session. While resting, I continued.)

D: Allow yourself to be surrounded by peace; allow yourself to grow stronger and stronger, day by day, and as you grow like the rose bush, with many flowers, the beautiful rose bush that you are, as you grow stronger and more passionate each day, allow yourself to move forward successfully in your life, to move forward successfully, financially and in every way. To be your own person, passionate and compassionate, and allow these feelings to grow stronger and stronger in you, as you move forward. As you move forward in a more positive way, you will see your excessive weight dripping off, pound by pound, as you become more passionate and successful, and you will feel better about yourself, more successful, more positive. The excessive weight will just keep dripping off pound by pound. Imagine now it already beginning, excess weight dripping off.

End of session.

As she came out of hypnosis, Madge looked peaceful and serene. She was very quiet, as though in a trance. "I have a lot to think about," she said. "One of the things I got from this session, I don't have to feel bad about or apologize for what I do or who I am."

It was now the first week in December. With her busy schedule and Christmas near, we set up the next appointment for the second week in January.

Session 3

I barely recognized Madge when she arrived. She was "effervescent." She greeted me with a big hug, smiling from ear to ear. She was now wearing makeup and wisps of her highlighted hair bounced around her face. Her beautiful cream-colored silk blouse peaked out from the light brown sweater thrown over her shoulders. She had a long floral skirt, slit on one side, which showed off her brown suede boots. She was radiant and full of life.

As we chatted, she said she had a new home address. Over the past month she found and moved into a condo that was light and airy, "where the sun can shine in the windows." Her next goal was to seek employment elsewhere. She joined Weight Watchers the beginning of January and was surprised to find out she had lost ten pounds over the holidays, "without even trying," she said. In this session, she wanted to go back to the time when she was nineteen years old. She became pregnant and remembers becoming panic-stricken. Was she still holding onto that energy?

She went easily into a deep hypnotic state and I age-regressed her:

D: You are now 19 years old. You learned you're pregnant. Panic has just set in, the panic of learning at nineteen years old you are pregnant. If you feel safe in doing so, allow yourself to enter into that state of panic.

M: My stomach, my lower stomach.

D: Go into your stomach. Go into the lower part of your stomach. Go into that feeling of panic. Just allow yourself to go deep into the panic and tell me what is going.

M: I just suddenly realized I'm pregnant. I spaced it out. I just – which is odd, because I always had so much trouble with my period. I should have recognized the fact that I hadn't had all the pain associated with my period every month. And – but I didn't have morning sickness or anything. I was two months, almost three months along before it dawned on me, or that I chose to recognize it. I started making bargains with God.

D: What were those bargains?

M: That I would raise somebody else's children. You know, I would take care of somebody else's kids.

D: And why would you do that?

M: Because I didn't want to have this baby. I didn't want to have the humiliation of knowing that the father didn't care anything about me, and the baby wouldn't know its father. I would be all alone and possibly stuck in the – I just didn't want the baby to go through everything I had gone through, and I just felt like that's what would end up happening to the baby, that we would never get out. We would never – that our lives would never be any better than it was right then. That I would never get away from the shame. (Speaking quietly.) That I would never get away from the shame.

D: Go into the shame. Go into the shame. Where is it?

M: (Deep breath.) I – the shame is (long pause).

D: Just allow yourself to feel it in your body. Where are you holding onto that shame? Allow it to come forth; go into the shame. Tell me where you are holding onto that shame.

M: I guess I – (Long pause.)

D: Just allow it to come forward; you can analyze it later. Allow it to come forward.

M: It – I often times don't look into people's faces when I pass them or when I talk to them. It's like I think they can see it in my eyes.

D: And what do they see?

M: That I made so many bad choices; that I was not strong enough. That's it, that I wasn't strong enough. I wanted so desperately to be loved, but I wasn't capable of loving the child I was carrying, because it was just something left over from a bad choice that I made.

D: That feeling. Where are you holding onto that feeling of not being capable of loving the child?

M: In my stomach.

D: Go back to your stomach. Go deep within your stomach.

M: It's like I carry evidence of that around with me.

D: Go into your stomach. Go deep within your stomach. Shrink yourself into a tiny, microscopic size, and go into your stomach and look around. What do you see?

M: I see this layer of fat, this layer of protection, because it's – it's just a layer of protection.

D: Now ask your Higher Self and your subconscious, is it is time to release the feeling of shame and guilt?

M: Yes, it is.

D: Imagine a magic toolbox with everything imaginable at your fingertips. Look at your toolbox. If you were to take something out of your toolbox to begin removing this feeling of shame and guilt in your stomach, what would you take out? What would you take out of your magic toolbox to being cutting out and removing this shame and the guilt that you have bestowed upon yourself?

M: Probably a pair of pliers.

D: Then take out your pliers. See them sparkle, nice and shiny pliers, and begin ripping out the shame and the guilt, removing all that darkness from your stomach. Begin ripping it out. And as you rip it out, allow it to flow down your legs and out your body onto the middle of the floor. Just remove it all and tear it out. Are you tearing it out?

M: Yes.

D: And how do you feel as you're tearing it out?

M: It's just black goo. Just kind of like oozing out like crude oil.

D: Just draining out your body?

M: Just draining out.

D: Good. Allow it to continue draining out, and as it drains out, allow the light to become brighter and brighter within. Allow the light to shine in and brighten the area. (Pause.) And when you are finished ripping everything out, look around and reach back into your magic toolbox for some healing water to rinse it out.

M: Just rinsing it out.

D: Cleanse it. Rinse everything so it's all sparkling, cleansed and healed.

D: And as you rinse it out, see the tissues in that area becoming healthier.

M: Yes, very healthy pink. Yeah!

D: Now look around. Is there anything else you would like to do before you leave that area?

M: No.

D: Now what would you like to fill that area with?

M: Just lots of love.

D: Then fill the area with love. What color would love represent to you?

M: It's a soft mauve color.

D: Allow the entire area to be filled with a soft mauve. A feeling of love for yourself and love for the children; love for the child that was there, knowing that at that time you were confused. You were alone. You were panicked. You were not ready to have a child to raise to adulthood. Fill the area with love and allow the love to penetrate throughout your body, knowing the choice you made at that time was the right choice for you.

M: Yes.

D: Now look around. Is there any guilt left?

M: No.

D: Have you cleansed yourself from all guilt and shame?
M: Yes.
D: Now go up to your face, your forehead, that area. Is there any shame left from that time?
M: Yes.
D: Where are you holding onto it?
M: In my jaw, my neck and my jaw.
D: Go into that area; go deep into that area. What does it say to you?
M: Hold your head up. It's okay. I'm okay.
D: Ask your Higher Self and your subconscious if it is time to remove the feeling of shame in the jaw and neck area.
M: Yes. Yes it is.
D: Then completely enclose it with a color. And what color would that be?
M: I think I will enclose it with pale green.
D: What would the color pale green, the feeling of shame, represent to you?
M: It represents, like an infection. It's just festered there.
D: It is time to remove the infection. Begin spitting it out your mouth.
M: Yeah.
D: Just get rid of it.
M: Just sucking it all out of there. Spitting it out. Suction it out.
D: All this time you have held onto it. It is now time to remove it.
M: Yes.
D: Is it all gone?
M: It is all gone.
D: And now, rinse the area out. Rinse the area out and cleanse it.
M: I'm gargling.
D: If you need to disinfect the area, go ahead.

M: Yes, the outside, and gargling, smiling in the mirror.

D: Try to remember that smile. Keep that smile on your face now that you have removed all the shame. And now, what would you like to fill that area with?

M: A rose color, soft rose color.

D: And what would that rose color represent?

M: Love and kindness, friendship.

D: Then allow yourself to fill the area with a rose color representing love, kindness, and friendship. Fill it totally and completely and feel it penetrating, penetrating all the cells in your jaw and neck area with love and kindness. Just allow it to be filled completely. And now go into your mind. Are you holding onto any negativity towards the removal of your pregnancy when you were nineteen? Are there any more negative thoughts towards that time?

M: Just my hips.

D: Then go into your hips; go into the hips. What are you holding onto in your hips? What does that represent?

M: It represents the burden. It represents burden. I think of my hips. It is burden.

D: Go into the burden, go into the feeling of the burden. What does that burden represent to you?

M: That I am supposed to be a mother. I'm supposed to want to have children. I don't, I don't want to have any children.

D: Go into the burden, then into the words "supposed to" that's implanted in the burden. Where did that come from, and why are you feeling you are "supposed to?"

M: My mother. My mother felt that they were a burden to her. She made me feel I was a burden. I didn't like the burden of having children. I had my brothers and sisters. I already had kids. I didn't want the responsibility of more children in my life. I already had kids.

D: Continue going deep into the feeling of the burden. Is there anything more? Allow it to come forward. Is there any more?

M: I wanted to be free of the burden. I wanted to be loved. I wanted to be encouraged. I wanted to grow and expand and I couldn't because I had the burden of all the children. I didn't want the burden of having kids of my own.

D: Ask your subconscious, your Higher Self, have you suffered enough through your lifetime with this burden? Is it time to remove it?

M: Yes it is, yes it is.

D: Then go into the feeling of the burden in your hips. Go into the feeling, the burden, the heavy weight of this burden, and what color would you give it?

M: Rusty brown.

D: And what does the rusty brown represent to you?

M: Just weight. It's sitting, weathered just like rusty steel or creosote-soaked wood, like ore, the color of ore.

D: It is time to remove it. Your subconscious and your Higher Self are removing this burden, this burden that has weighed so heavily upon your body for so many years. Take this rusty brown color, the color of ore and begin pushing it down your legs, pushing it out your toes. Cut it away if you need to. Go into your magic toolbox. Whatever you need to remove it is in your toolbox.

M: Yeah, just chiseling it off. Just breaking it and it just falls away.

D: Continue doing that. It is time to remove it.

M: Yeah. (Pause.) It's nice. The skin underneath is beautiful, white, milky-smooth skin.

D: Have you chipped it all away?

M: Yeah. I'm starting to work on the right one now.

D: Continue. Take your time. Let me know when you're finished.

M: (Pause, then deep sigh.) It's all chipped away.

D: And now cleanse the entire area with cool, clear, healing water. Rinse it all off and see the beautiful white, milky-smooth skin underneath.

M: Yes.

D: Soft, gentle skin, healthy skin, healthy skin underneath. You have carried the burden far too long.

M: Yes.

D: It is now washed away and cleansed. What would you like to seal the beautiful skin with? You have removed the burden; now seal the beautiful skin.

M: I'm putting on this balm. I'm rubbing on this balm on my hips, this balm that is full of this love, this healing love! Just smoothing it and sealing it all up, just rubbing it on my legs and my hips. (Pause.) That looks good. That feels good. Makes everything like it's supposed to, like it's supposed to really be.

D: Let me know when you're finished.

M: It doesn't bother her anymore.

D: And who is her?

M: Me, her is me, her is me.

D: Allow yourself to become one. Allow yourself to become one with yourself. See yourself integrating her and me to become one. Are you doing that?

M: Yes, I did. It's funny! She's standing there and I'm standing there looking at – it's almost like one person walked into another person's body. I'm standing there looking at my arms and my hands and it's comfortable. It doesn't feel foreign at all. I don't feel like it's a person that has to hide away, a person that always has to make sure that nobody knew.

D: See yourself as you truly are. Look at yourself. Look at yourself and see the real you, the true you, the true you that you are, the you who you are now allowing yourself to be. Take your time and look at yourself, and enjoy yourself.

M: Yes. She – she's excited! And when I see my face now, I see reflections of her in me. I have a light in me that wasn't there before.

D: Allow this light to grow stronger and stronger each passing day. Allow your light to grow stronger. And now, as you look at yourself and realize your full potential, check your body inside and out. Is there any other area that needs attention?

M: My upper arms.

D: Go into your upper arms. Go into your upper arms and your shoulders. What are you feeling?

M: There's – she's in there, being held is foreign to her. I don't recognize this person. It's me, but I don't recognize her.

D: And how do you see her?

M: She's so dark. She's so sad.

D: Is that the former you?

M: Yes.

D: Is it time to (Marge abruptly interrupts.)

M: (Loud voice.) This person! It's time for this person to leave. It's like the person is in spirit and not physical.

D: Give her a big hug because she has been a part of you and she has helped you.

M: Yeah, she has.

D: Just give her a big hug and then send her away with love. It is time for her to leave, for the new you to take over.

M: Yes, yes it is. She's being – like angels. She has a pair of wings on. She was crying. She was sitting on a chair in a dark room and she was crying because of the loneliness. She has her face in her hands.

D: Tell her goodbye and that you will be okay. You no longer need her. The light is growing stronger within you now. You no longer need her. It is time to release her.

M: I took out scissors from my toolbox and cut the connection. The cord is cut.

D: Then allow her to be released and seal up the area where the cord was cut. Just seal it up.

M: Ooohhh, this silver, this beautiful silver light that is around her. The cord was cut. She's excited about the fact that she – when I left, she wanted to be held. She wanted to be rocked like a child. Being touched won't be uncomfortable for me – have someone hold me. It will be natural. It will feel normal, and the spirit part that left is looking hopeful and expectant of good things. She's kind of apart, almost like that part of her is just gone to spirit now and it's okay, it's okay.

D: Is she gone now?

M: That part that left, the part that she cut the cord on, it went to – the spirit went up, the spirit went up, separate.

D: And now go back into your shoulder. Shrink yourself down and look around in your shoulders. Imagine yourself microscopic. Look around. What do you see?

M: I see this beautiful, small, smooth shoulder.

D: Is there anything else you need to do to the shoulders?

M: No. The shoulder is good. The shoulder is very good.

D: Is the pain removed?

M: The pain is removed.

D: Is the negativity gone?

M: The negativity is gone. It's a beautiful shoulder. It is very healthy, very smooth, very strong.

D: Is there anything you would like to do to keep this area healthy?

M: (Pause.) There's this positive golden light that just kind of emanates from the bones, that just generates this beautiful warm healing, and it's just very healthy.

D: Allow it to grow stronger and stronger. (Pause.) And now, go back into your brain. Go back into your brain and see if there is any other part of your body that needs attention.

M: Let's see. (Long pause.)

D: Is there any other part of your body that needs attention? Scan your body. Ask your brain, your Higher Self, your subconscious, is there is any other part of your body that needs attention?

M: Her sadness will not be there as much. She will, she'll find her growth, her path, her reason for being here. She'll be able to accomplish it. She's been lifting my face. I am me. I am she. I am lifting my face more. I am opening my eyes and looking at things. And things that I look at can't harm me because I am not afraid of there being shame in my eyes because there isn't anymore. The shame isn't in my eyes anymore.

D: Is there anything else that you need to deal with at this time? Ask your subconscious and your Higher Self if there is anything else you need to deal with at this time. Allow it to come forward.

M: Yeah. I need to deal with the fact that Edward may not love me. He – in a past life – in love. I may have to go on in this life without him.

D: Then you understand this and accept it. Know that there are other loves from your past and there may be a different love in this lifetime.

M: Yes.

D: It is not anything you have to worry about at this time.

M: No.

D: Just know that you are bringing forth yourself. You are bringing forth the love for yourself at this (Madge interrupts.)

M: Yes! Yes I am. I am bringing forth the love for myself in this lifetime. Yes. It is so much lighter with all the pain gone. It's like there was so much burden; it's gone away. I wanted to be a good person. I didn't want to hurt anyone, but I gave so much of myself when I was doing that.

D: You know within yourself you are a very good person. You know that.

M: Yes.

D: All the things you went through in your childhood and in your life, you gave up yourself. You have now come back to be the person, to be the person you truly are. You never intentionally hurt someone. There are many things that you have had to deal with in your lifetime. Sometimes they place confusion and panic within us.

M: Yes, yes.

D: And have you removed that? And now are you in control of yourself and your choices?

M: Yes.

D: You are now in control of yourself and your choices. You have released the negativity and you are now allowing yourself to be open to the happiness that you deserve.

M: Yes. I have.

D: The happiness is there for you. Allow it to come into your life. Know it will be there.

M: Yes, it will be. She – I have a light about me that I didn't see before. Other people see it, but I haven't seen it before.

D: And where is the light?

M: It's like all around me, like, it's like being shown down upon, but it's emanating from me at the same time. She's healing. I'm getting the love back that (long pause).

D: Tell me what's going on?

M: Being able to love someone. Being able to be loving toward someone, and still know when that person doesn't have your best interest is okay. Kindness is an everyday activity. Kindness is something to do without giving yourself away. You can be kind, and taking care of yourself is not selfish. She was always, I was always afraid that I was being selfish, that I wasn't giving enough, and if I gave more I would be loved. But that wasn't right. She had the idea, she just had it turned around.

D: Is there any other place you need to go that is unfinished?

M: No.

(Madge was guided to her peaceful place, where she rested and re-energized.)

End of session.

As a child, Madge had the mistaken belief that because she enjoyed touching people, feeling their skin, it was her fault her uncle continually molested her. Aunt Anna loved her niece, but because of her constantly verbalizing her distain for womanhood and her husband who was physically violent and emotionally abusive, Madge became subconsciously programmed to not want to be a woman. This came out in her later years in the way she dressed, acted, and kept herself physically. Her excess weight was a protective device to not attract men, "If I'm not pretty, men won't be attracted to me."

Madge had many years of emotional and physical pain she had been carrying around, like a wagon full of bricks dragging behind her. With the removal of this "baggage," she was beautiful and glowing, like a caterpillar that had just come out of its cocoon and was transformed into a beautiful butterfly, dancing in the spring air. As she left my office, my thoughts were, "her life is just beginning."

If there is light in the soul,
There will be beauty in the person.
If there is beauty in the person,
There will be harmony in the house.
If there is harmony in the house,
There will be order in the nation,
There will be peace in the world.

— Chinese proverb

Chapter 9

Conclusion

When a person is hypnotized, it may appear that he is reliving a past lifetime where his body and mind seem to re-experience traumatic, as well as positive events, even recognizing others from the past brought forth into the present. Still under hypnosis, it may appear he is going to the other side, prior to being born, and at times taken into the future, all while sitting in a reclining chair in my office. Does this indicate time is linear? Does this indicate reality or is the client's subconscious creating a believable story for the self? Will past lives someday be scientifically proven? Only time will tell.

Although we may have had many past lives and may be able to access "the other side," what really matters is NOW, living in the present. Perhaps this is why we have been given techniques that access these areas in order to heal current issues and allow a person to function optimally in the present. Living in the moment is most important, not living in the past. Our past experiences help us to become who we are, just as what happened yesterday affects us today. We learn from our past so we may move forward with balance and harmony in our future.

I have shared with you a variety of cases and their outcomes, which are some of the many ways hypnosis supports people's freedom, growth, and joy. Isn't it time to rid yourself of physical ailments that are no longer useful, as in the case of Esther who had a continual pain in her neck and shoulder, or Evelyn with a hip misalignment, now no longer requiring the help of a chiropractor for leg adjustments, and Henry who previously suffered from chronic shoulder pain for years? In the cases of Elena and Joanne, migraine headaches stopped once the original cause was identified and understood. Sandy had been persecuted for her gifts of physic abilities, those gifts to be enhanced once the guilt from her past was removed. With Madge, removing ethereal pounds she had been carrying around for many years led to the removal of physical pounds, resulting in the transformation to the beautiful person she truly is instead of the person her inner guilt had caused her to become.

By clearing those issues that cling to us, holding us back, we can love and be loved for the right reasons, not because we need to be with a mate or loved one, but because we want to be with a mate or loved one. It is said we draw to us what we put out, so decide now to free yourself from old energies that bind you and make your life the best that it can be.

God is love, and if we are made in God's image, we are made of love, a wonderful energy of strength and beauty. When you love yourself, you obtain a spiritual peace and sense of calmness within, and you shine that energy on others. You have such a great opportunity to make changes in your life and to learn more about your total person, who you really are in all dimensions.

Working with my clients has enhanced and enriched my life. There are so many caring people in the world who are quietly crying out, and the use of hypnosis is a cutting-edge healing modality available to all with no pins, needles, or medications needed to obtain optimal freedom from within.

May you walk unencumbered in the light and love of God.

Bibliography

Baldwin, William. (1992). *Spirit Releasement Therapy: A Technique Manual.* (2nd ed.). Terra Alta, WV: Headline Books.

Baldwin, William. (1999). CE-VI: *Close Encounters of the Possession Kind.* Terra Alta, WV: Headline Books, Inc.

Bandler, R., and Grinder, J. (1982). *Reframing: Neuro-Linguistic Programming and the Transformation of Meaning.* Moab, UT: Real People Press.

Barber, Joseph. (1996). *Hypnosis and Suggestion in the Treatment of Pain.* (1st ed.). New York, NY: W. W. Norton & Company, Inc.

Blakemore, Colin. (1977). *Mechanics of the Mind.* Cambridge: Cambridge University Press.

Bletzer, June G. (1986). *The Encyclopedic Psychic Dictionary.* Lithia Springs, GA: New Leaf Distributing Company.

Bowman, Carol. (1997). *Children's Past Lives: How Past Life Memories Affect Your Child.* New York: Bantam.

Burnham, Sophy. (1990). *A Book of Angels: Reflections on Angels Past- Present - True Stores of How They Touch Our Lives.* New York: Ballantine.

Cannon, Dolores. (2001). *They Walked with Jesus: Past Life Experiences with Christ.* AR: Ozark Mountain Publishers.

Cayce, Hugh Lynn. (1967). *Edgar Cayce on Reincarnation.* VA: The Association for Research and Enlightenment.

Chopra, Deepak. (1989). *Quantum Healing.* New York: Bantam.

Cousins, Norman. (1979). *Anatomy of an Illness as Perceived by the Patient.* New York: Bantam.

Davis, L.W. and Husband, R.W., "Hypnotic Suggestibility in Relation to Personality Traits". *Journal of Abnormal and Social Psychology,* 26:175, 1931.

Dossey, Larry. (1989). *Recovering the Soul: A Scientific and Spiritual Search.* New York: Bantam.

Ellenberger, Henri F. (1970). T*he Discovery of the Unconscious.* New York: Basic Books.

Erickson, Milton H. (Jay Haley, ed.) (1967). *Advanced Techniques of Hypnosis and Therapy.* Grune & Stratton, Inc.: New York and London.

Erickson, M.E. and E.L. Rossi. (1981). *Experiencing Hypnosis: Therapeutic Approaches to Altered States.* New York: Irvington Publishers.

Fiore, Edith. (1978). *You Have Been Here Before.* New York: Ballantine.

Fiore, Edith. (1989). *Encounters.* New York: Doubleday.

Fischer, Joe. (1985). *The Case for Reincarnation.* New York: Bantam Books.

Foulks, E. (1985). In B. O'Regan (Ed.), *Investigations:* Research Bulletin of the Institute of Noetic Sciences. Vol. 1, No. ¾ (p. 7). Sausalito, CA: IONS.

Frejer, B. Ernest. (1995). *The Edgar Cayce Companion: A Comprehensive Treatise of the Edgar Cayce Readings.* Virginia Beach, VA: A.R.E. Press.

Gabriel, Michael. (1992). *Voices From The Womb.* Lower Lake, CA: Aslan.

Gardner, G. G., and K. Olness. (1981) *Hypnosis and Hypnotherapy with Children.* Orlando: Grune & Stratton.

Gawain, Shakti. (1978). *Creative Visualization.* Mill Valley, CA: Whatever Publishing.

Gordon, David and Meyers-Anderson, Maribeth. (1981). *Phoenix: Therapeutic Patterns of Milton H. Erickson.* Cupertino, CA: Meta Publications.

Grinder, J. and Bandler, R. (1981). *Trance-formations: Neuro-Linguistic Programming and the Structure of Hypnosis.* Real People Press: Moab, UT.

Grof, Stan. (1975). *Realms of the Human Unconscious: Observations from LSD Research.* New York: Viking Press.

Grof, Stan. (1985). *Beyond The Brain.* New York: State University of New York.

Hammond, D. (Ed.). (1990). *Handbook of Hypnotic Suggestions and Metaphors.* An American Society of Clinical Hypnosis Book. New York: W.W. Norton & Co.

Head and V. Cranston (1977). *Reincarnation: The Phoenix Fire Mysteries.* New York: Julian.

Henderson, Charles E. (1983). *You Can Do It With Self Hypnosis.* Englewood Cliffs, NJ: Prentice-Hall.

Hickman, Irene. (1983). *Mind Probe – Hypnosis.* Kirksville, MO: Hickman Systems.

Hilgard, Ernest R. and Josephine R. (1975). *Hypnosis and the Relief of Pain.* Los Altos, CA: William Kaufmann.

Hodson, G. (1967). *Reincarnation: Fact or Fallacy.* Wheaton, IL: The Theosophical Publishing House.

Ingerman, Sandra. (1991). *Soul Retrieval.* San Francisco: Harper.

James, Tad & Woodsmall, Wyatt. (1988). *Time Line Therapy: And The Basis of Personality.* Capitola, CA: Meta Publications

Kelsey, Denys and Grant, Joan. (1987). *Many Lifetimes.* New York: Ballantine.

Korn, E. R. (1983). *Visualization: Use of Imagery in the Health Professions.* Homewood, IL: Dow Jones-Irwin.

Krasner, A.M. (1990/1991). *The Wizard Within: The Krasner Method of Hypnotherapy.* Santa Ana, CA: American Board of Hypnotherapy Press.

Kroger, William S. (1977). *Clinical and Experimental Hypnosis* (2nd ed.). Philadelphia: Lippincott.

Kubler-Ross, Elizabeth. (1969). *On Death and Dying.* New York: MacMillan.

Lucas, Winafred Blake. (1993). *Regression Therapy: A Handbook for Professionals —Volume I: Past-Life Therapy.* Crest Park, CA: Deep Forest Press.

Lucas, Winafred Blake. (1993). *Regression Therapy: A Handbook for Professionals- Volume II: Special Instances of Altered State Work.* Crest Park, CA: Deep Forest Press.

Mills, J.C., and R. .J. Crowley. (1986). *Therapeutic Metaphors for the Child Within.* New York: Brunner/Mazel, Inc.

Montgomery, Ruth. (1985). *Aliens Among Us.* New York, NY: Ballantine.

Montgomery, Ruth. (1979). *Strangers Among Us.* New York: Ballantine.

Moody, Raymond A. (1990). *Coming Back: A Psychiatrist Explores Past-Life Journeys.* New York: Bantam, Doubleday, Dell Publishing Group.

Myss, Caroline. (2002). *Sacred Contracts: Awakening Your Divine Potential.* New York: Three Rivers Press.

Netherton, Morris and Shiffrin, Nancy. (1978). *Past Lives Therapy.* New York: Ace Books.

Newton, Michael. (1994). *Journey of Souls: Case Studies of Life Between Lives.* (5th ed.) St. Paul, MN: Llewellyn Publications.

Newton, Michael. (2000). *Destiny of Souls: New Case Studies of Life Between Lives.* St. Paul, MN: Llewellyn Publications.

Oppenheim, Garrett. (1990). *Who Were You Before You Were You?* New York: Carlton Press.

Ostrom, Joseph. (1987). *You and Your Aura.* Wellingborough, Northamptonshire, Great Britain: The Aquarian Press.

Pelletier, K. R. (1977). *Mind as Healer, Mind as Slayer.* New York: Dell.

Rawat, K. S. (1986). *Venture Inward, Premier Issue.* Interview with Dr. Ian Stevenson. Fairdabad, India: Reincarnation Research Foundation.

Restak, Richard. (1984). *The Brain.* New York: Bantam.

Ross, Colin. (1989). *Multiple Personality:Diagnosis, Clinical Features and Treatment.* New York: Wiley.

Rossetti, Francesca. (1992). *Psycho Regression: A New System for Healing & Personal Growth.* London: Judy Piatkus (Publishers).

Samuels, M., and Samuels, N. (1975). *Seeing with the Mind's Eye.* New York: Random House.

Schlotterbeck, Karl. (1987). *Living Your Past Lives: The Psychology of Past-Life Regression.* New York: Ballantine.

Shealy, Norman and Myss, Caroline. (1988). *The Creation of Health: The Emotional, Psychological, and Spiritual Responses That Promote Health and Healing.* New York: Three Rivers.

Sutphen, Dick. (1976). *You Were Born Again To Be Together.* New York: Simon & Schuster.

Verney, Thomas. (1982). *The Secret Life of the Unborn Child.* New York: Dell.

Wambach, Helen. (1978). *Reliving Past Lives.* New York: Harper & Row.

Wambach, Helen. (1979). *Life Before Life.* New York: Wm. Morrow.

Weiss, Brian. (1988). *Many Lives, Many Masters.* New York: Simon & Schuster.

Weiss, Brian. (1993). *Through Time into Healing: Discovering the Power of Regression Therapy to Erase Trauma and Transform Mind, Body, and Relationships.* New York: Touchstone.

Wester, W., and Smith, A. (1984). *Clinical Hypnosis.* New York: J. B. Lippincott.

White Eagle Publishing Trust. (2000). *Jesus Teacher and Healer, from White Eagle's Teaching.* (2nd ed.) Great Britain: University Press.

Whitfield, Charles. (1987). *Healing the Child Within.* Deerfield Beach, FL: Health Communications.

Whitton, Joel, & Fisher, Joe. (1986). *Life Between Life.* New York: Doubleday.

Williston, G. and Johnstone, J. (1983). *Discovering Your Past Lives.* Northampton, England: Thorsons Publishing Group.

Wolberg, Lewis R. (1972). *Hypnosis: Is It For You?* New York: Harcourt, Brace, Jovanovich.

Wolf, F.A. (1981.) *Taking the Quantum Leap.* New York: Harper and Row.

Woolger, Roger. (1987). *Other Lives, Other Selves: A Jungian Psychotherapist Discovers Past Lives.* New York: Doubleday.

Wyckoff, James. (1975). *Franz Mesmer: Between God and the Devil.* London: Prentice-Hall.

IF YOU LIKED THIS BOOK, YOU WON'T WANT TO MISS

OTHER TITLES BY DANDELION BOOKS

Available Now And Always Through www.dandelionbooks.net And Affiliated Websites!!

TOLL-FREE ORDERS – 1-800-861-7899 (U.S. & CANADA)

Non-Fiction - Conscious Solutions:

Living with Soul: An Old Soul's Guide to Life, the Universe and Everything, Vol. I, by Tony Stubbs... Who are we? Where did we come from? Why are we here? Master teacher and sage Tony Stubbs urges us to "go to the Source... look in the mirror." In the first of a two-volume compendium of comprehensive spiritual teachings, Stubbs expertly documents his lessons and observations with excellent anecdotes, charts and other graphics. (ISBN 1-893302-85-7)

Living with Soul: An Old Soul's Guide to Life, the Universe and Everything, Vol. II, by Tony Stubbs... Learn how to work with energy and make it work for you by discovering your own energy patterns or bio-rhythms. Explore reincarnation, death, grief, near-death experiences, life on the "other side" and many other multi-dimensional experiences. Also learn more about the coming U.S. disclosures concerning extraterrestrials, UFOs and many cover-ups that may have "Earth-shattering" repercussions for those who until now have been unwilling to accept that "we are not alone." (ISBN 1-893302-86-5)

Portals to Higher Consciousness: Exploring the Spiritual Domain, by Norman D. Livergood... What is the process that serious students use to actually realize—bring to manifestation—their Higher Consciousness, "through which they are able to contact Reality in a region of pure Truth." If you're interested in investigating higher consciousness, put on your hiking clothes and join this spiritual expedition (1-893302-92X)

Creation and Metempsychosis (The Evolution of the Soul): An Introduction to the "Psychological Key of Man," edited and compiled by Q. Dean Sloan... A compilation of theosophical metaphysics that provides the technical metaphysical rationale for Creation itself, as well as Creation of the human soul ("crown chakra") and is based on the psychology of the 7 rays. "The 'petals' in the crown chakra unfold slowly over a long series of lives, and we achieve perfection only when they have completely unfolded." (ISBN 1-893302-90-7)

The Perennial Tradition: Overview Of The Secret Heritage, The Single Stream Of Initiatory Teaching Flowing Through All The Great Schools Of Mysticism, by Norman D. Livergood... Like America, Awake, this book is another wake-up call. "It was written to assist readers to awaken to the Higher Spiritual World." In addition to providing a history of the Western tradition of the Perennial Tradition, Livergood also describes the process that serious students use to actually realize–bring to manifestation–their Higher Consciousness. "Unless we become aware of this higher state, we face the prospect of a basically useless physical existence and a future life–following physical death–of unpleasant, perhaps anguished reformation of our essence." (ISBN 1-893302-48-2)

Progressive Awareness: Critical Thinking, Self-Awareness & Critical Consciousness, by Norman D. Livergood... how to avoid being manipulated by our emotions and ideas and how to start thinking for ourselves; increase your skills for understanding, critical thinking, self-awareness, critical consciousness, and enlightened discernment. (ISBN 1-893302-80-6)

My Name is Esther Clara, by Laurel Johnson... Esther Clara's lifetime spanned two world wars and the inventions of electricity, telephones, automobiles, airplanes, radio, TV, computers and many other conveniences that have become basic necessities of modern American life. An authentic first-hand account of 20th Century rural America audio and videotaped before her death and adeptly reconstituted by master storyteller and book reviewer, Laurel Johnson. (ISBN 1-893302-89-X)

Why Don't You Love Me? I'm the Best Choice: Repairing Heartache, Finding the Right Mate & Not Making the Same Mistakes the Next Time, by Debi Davis... Everyone has a perfect mate waiting for them and it may not be the person you are trying to hold onto now. Learn how to manifest that perfect partner... for you by clearly identifying the qualities you're looking for and making sure you show the world a true and honest portrait of who you are. (ISBN 1-893302-91-1)

The Compassionate Surgeon, by Joop Schokker, M.D. . . . Do you or someone you love need an operation? Scared? Don't know where to turn for advice? Let Dr. Joop Schokker guide you through the process and answer such questions as: What should you expect before, during and after surgery? What should you ask of, and expect from, your surgeon? What can go wrong and how will your surgeon fix it? When is surgery unnecessary? What are your chances of full recovery? (ISBN 0-963294-76-8)

Executive Parenting: Risks & Solutions for the Working Parent- What you may not know . . . but will wish you did!, by Debi Davis & Ellen Sherman, Ph.D....Health expert Debi Davis and Marriage and Family Counselor Dr. Ellen Sherman have combined their knowledge and experience to deliver a comprehensive manual for child-rearing in the 21st century. (ISBN 1-893302-93-8)

The Courage To Be Who I Am, by Mary-Margareht Rose... This book is rich with teachings and anecdotes delivered with humor and humanness, by a woman who followed her heart and learned to listen to her inner voice; in the process, transforming every obstacle into an opportunity to test her courage to manifest her true identity. (1SBN 1-893302-13-X)

The Making Of A Master: Tracking Your Self-Worth, by Jeanette O'Donnal... A simple tracking method for self-improvement that takes the mystery out of defining your goals, making a road map and tracking your progress. A book rich with nuggets of wisdom couched in anecdotes and instructive dialogues. (ISBN 1-893302-36-9)

Fiction with Flare:

Waaaay Out There! Diggertown, Oklahoma, by Tuklo Nashoba...Adventures of constable Clint Mankiller and his deputy, Chad GhostWolf; Jim Bob and Bubba Johnson, Grandfather GhostWolf, Cassie Snodgrass, Doc Jones, Judge Jenkins and the rest of the Diggertown, Oklahoma bunch in the first of a series of Big Foot-Sasquatch tall tales peppered with lots of good belly laughs and just as much fun. (ISBN 1-893302-44-X)

Waaaay Out There! Arbuckle Treasure Hunt, by Tuklo Nashoba... The second in the WAAAAY OUT THERE series that takes Clint Mankiller and his deputy, Chad GhostWolf, Bubba and the rest of the Diggertown gang high up in to the Arbuckle Mountains on a hunt for buried Spanish gold. Maps, hidden chests and dangerous Werewolves are all part of the adventure that even manages to turn up the old man who originally buried the gold! Buckle up for some more great laughs and lots of campfire fun. (ISBN 1-893302-65-2)

Drifters: The Final Testament, Volume One, by Michael Silverhawk... Within the DRIFTERS trilogy is a powerful secret, a key that unlocks our human potential! Can one man "make a difference" not only in his own life but for everyone else on the planet? Is it possible for a single human to transform chaos into order, darkness into light? (ISBN 1-893302-57-1)

Ticket to Paradise, by Yvonne Ridley...Judith Tempest, a British reporter, is searching for the Truth. But when it starts to spill out in her brilliant front page reportage of Middle East suicide bombing in retaliation for Israeli tanks mowing down innocent Palestinian women and children, both 'Tempest' and 'Truth' start to spell 'Trouble'– with a capital 'T', joke her friends and colleagues. A non-stop mystery thriller that tears along at a reckless pace of passion, betrayal, adventure and espionage. (ISBN 1-893302-77-6)

Synchronicity Gates: An Anthology Of Stories And Poetry About People Transformed In Extraordinary Reality Beyond Experience, by Stephen Vernarelli... An inventive compilation of short stories that take the reader beyond mere science, fiction, or fantasy. Vernarelli introduces the reader to a new perception of reality; he imagines the best and makes it real. (ISBN 1-893302-38-5)

The Alley of Wishes, by Laurel Johnson... Despite the ravages of WWI on Paris and on the young American farm boy, Beck Sanow, and despite the abusive relationship that the chanteuse Cerise endures, the two share a bond that is unbreakable by time, war, loss of memory, loss of life and loss of youth. Beck and Cerise are both good people beset by constant tragedy. Yet it is tragedy that brings them together, and it is unconditional love that keeps them together. (ISBN 1-893302-46-6)

Freedom: Letting Go Of Anxiety And Fear Of The Unknown, by Jim Britt... Jeremy Carter, a fireman from Missouri who is in New York City for the day, decides to take a tour of the Trade Center, only to watch in shock, the attack on its twin towers from a block away. Afterward as he gazes at the pit of rubble and talks with many of the survivors, Jeremy starts to explore the inner depths of his soul, to ask questions he'd never asked before. This dialogue helps him learn who he is and what it takes to overcome the fear, anger, grief and anxiety this kind of tragedy brings. (ISBN 1-893302-74-1)

The Prince Must Die, by Gower Leconfield... breaks all taboos for mystery thrillers. After the "powers that be" suppressed the manuscripts of three major British writers, Dandelion Books breaks through with a thriller involving a plot to assassinate Prince Charles. The Prince Must Die brings to life a Britain of today that is on the edge with race riots, neo-Nazis, hard right backlash and neo-punk nihilists. Riveting entertainment... you won't be able to put it down. (ISBN 1-893302-72-5)

Come as You Are, by Sarah Daniels... "Tongue-in-cheek" entertainment at its wackiest—and most subtle. If anyone ever doubted that sex makes the world go around, author Sarah Daniels will put your mind, and body to test. Non-stop humor, humanness and wisdom are bundled together to deliver one of life's most important unheeded lessons: each of us has a unique destiny to discover, and until we find and embark on that destiny, life may be one bowl of cherry pits after another. Adult language and scenes. (ISBN 1-893302-15-6)

Unfinished Business, by Elizabeth Lucas Taylor... Lindsay Mayer knows something is amiss when her husband, Griffin, a college professor, starts spending too much time at his office and out-of-town. Shortly after the ugly truth surfaces, Griffin disappears altogether. Lindsay is shattered. Life without Griffin is life without life... One of the sexiest books you'll ever read! (ISBN 1-893302-68-7)

The Woman With Qualities, by Sarah Daniels... South Florida isn't exactly the Promised Land that forty-nine-year-old newly widowed Keri Anders had in mind when she transplanted herself here from the northeast... A tough action-packed novel that is far more than a love story. (ISBN 1-893302-11-3)

Adventure Capital, by John Rushing...South Florida adventure, crime and violence in a fiction story based on a true life experience. A book you will not want to put down until you reach the last page. (ISBN 1-893302-08-3)

A Mother's Journey: To Release Sorrow And Reap Joy, by Sharon Kay... A poignant account of Norah Ann Mason's life journey as a wife, mother and single parent. This book will have a powerful impact on anyone, female or male, who has experienced parental abuse, family separations, financial struggles and a desperate need to find the magic in life that others talk about that just doesn't seem to be there for them. (ISBN 1-893302-52-0)

Return To Masada, by Robert G. Makin... In a gripping account of the famous Battle of Masada, Robert G. Makin skillfully recaptures the blood and gore as well as the spiritual essence of this historic struggle for freedom and independence. (ISBN 1-893302-10-5)

Time Out Of Mind, by Solara Vayanian... Atlantis had become a snake pit of intrigue teeming with factious groups vying for power and control. An unforgettable drama that tells of the breakdown of the priesthood, the hidden scientific experiments in genetic engineering which produced "things" – part human and part animal – and other atrocities; the infiltration by the dark lords of Orion; and the implantation of the human body with a device to fuel the Orion wars. (ISBN 1-893302-21-0)

The Thirteenth Disciple: The Life Of Mary Magdalene, by Gordon Thomas... The closest of Jesus' followers, the name of Mary Magdalene conjures images of a woman both passionate and devoted, both sinner and saint. The first full-length biography for 13 centuries. (ISBN 1-893302-17-2)

Non-Fiction – Uncensored and Unfettered:

Adam & Evil: The God Who hates Sex, Women and Human Bodies, by The Heyeokah Guru . . . EXPOSED: 'Jesus Christ' is a mythological figure, not a person. The Virgin Mary is the Earth, not a young woman who never had sex; Heaven and Hell are right here! We create them ourselves. The truth at last about one of the greatest conspiracies in the world! (ISBN 1-893302-94-6)

It's All about Control: The God, Jesus and ET Cover-up Conspiracies, by Tony Stubbs... Three major conspiracies are controlling the people of planet Earth: This book provides the truth-serum and tools for breaking free from a cruel, cleverly contrived mind-control game that for centuries has been keeping the human race in bondage to the Religion, War and Finance industries. (ISBN 1-893302-95-4)

The Host & The Parasite: How Israel's Fifth Column Consumed America, by Greg Felton... "The United States became midwife to a war crime when it endorsed the creation of Israel in 1948 and blackmailed European nations into supporting it," writes Felton. "From this time forward, the Zionist parasite began leaching off the U.S." A definitive study of "Israel's conquest of America and its use of the U.S. economy, government and military to terrorize the Muslim world." (ISBN 1-893302-99-7)

Tracking Deception: Bush Mid-East Policy, by William A. Cook... "Bill Cook writes with vivid urgency as he excavates the Augean muck of the Bush years, subjecting the president and his gang to an excruciatingly tight close-up, where every flaw, every imperfection, every touch-up is exposed to all who dare to look."—Alex Cockburn, Counterpunch Editor-in-Chief [from the Introduction] (ISBN 1-893302-83-0)

Exopolitics: Political Implications Of The Extraterrestrial Presence, by Michael E. Salla, Ph.D.... According to Dr. Michael Salla and many other experts in the field of ET research, for almost 70 years the US government has engaged in an extensive "official effort" of disinformation, intimidation and tampering with evidence in order to maintain a non-disclosure policy about extraterrestrial presence. (ISBN 1-893302-56-3)

America Speaks Out: Collected Essays From Dissident Writers John H. Brand, Meria Heller, John Kaminski, Norman D. Livergood, Wayne Madsen, Kurt Nimmo, Albert D. Pastore, Michael E. Salla, Sherman H. Skolnick & John Stanton... A collection of essays extracted from works recently published by Dandelion Books. (ISBN 1-893302-63-6)

America 2004: A Power But Not Super, by John Stanton [Foreword by Bev Conover, Editor - onlinejournal.com, Introduction by Karen Kwiatkowski, Lieutenant Colonel, USAF (Ret.)]... Stanton explains how Bush has adroitly fused state, religious (faith-based government) and business interests into one indistinguishable tyrannical mass... his explanation of how this has been accomplished is eye-opening. (ISBN 1-893302-26-1)

Stranger than Fiction: An Independent Investigation Of The True Culprits Behind 9-11, by Albert D. Pastore, Ph.D... Twelve months of careful study, painstaking research, detailed analysis, source verification and logical deduction went into the writing of this book. In addition to the stories are approximately 300 detailed footnotes. Pastore: "Only by sifting through huge amounts of news data on a daily basis was I able to catch many of these rare 'diamonds in the rough' and organize them into a coherent pattern and logical argument." (ISBN 1-893302-47-4)

Unshackled: A Survivor's Story of Mind Control, by Kathleen Sullivan... A non-fictional account of Kathleen Sullivan's experiences as part of a criminal network that includes Intelligence personnel, military personnel, doctors and mental health professionals contracted by the military and the CIA, criminal cult leaders and members, pedophiles, pornographers, drug dealers and Nazis. "I believe my story needs to be told so that more people will understand how 'Manchurian Candidate' style mind-control techniques can create alter-states in the minds of unwitting victims, causing them to perform deeds that are normally repugnant." (ISBN 1-893302-35-0)

Ahead Of The Parade: A Who's Who Of Treason and High Crimes – Exclusive Details Of Fraud And Corruption Of The Monopoly Press, The Banks, The Bench And The Bar, And The Secret Political Police, by Sherman H. Skolnick... One of America's foremost investigative reporters, speaks out on some of America's current crises. Included in this blockbuster book are the following articles: Big City Newspapers & the Mob, The Sucker Traps, Dirty Tricks of Finance and Brokerage, The Secret History of Airplane Sabotage, Wal-Mart and the Red Chinese Secret Police, The Chandra Levy Affair, The Japanese Mafia in the United States, The Secrets of Timothy McVeigh, and much more. (ISBN 1-893302-32-6)

Another Day in The Empire: Life in Neoconservative America, by Kurt Nimmo... A collection of articles by one of Counterpunch's most popular columnists. Included in this collection are: The Son of COINTELPRO; Clueless at the State Department; Bush Senior: Hating Saddam, Selling Him Weapons; Corporate Media: Selling Dubya's Oil War; Iraq and the Vision of the Velociraptors: The Bleeding Edge of Islam; Condoleezza Rice at the Waldorf Astoria; Predators, Snipers and the Posse Comitatus Act, and many others.

Palestine & The Middle East: Passion, Power & Politics, by Jaffer Ali... The Palestinian struggle is actually a human one that transcends Palestine... There is no longer a place for Zionism in the 20th century... Democracy in the Middle East is not safe for US interests as long as there is an atmosphere of hostility... Suicide bombings are acts of desperation and mean that a people have been pushed to the brink... failure to understand why they happen will make certain they will continue. Jaffer Ali is a Palestinian-American business man who has been writing on politics and business for over 25 years. (ISBN 1-893302-45-8)

Ben-Gurion's Scandals: How The Haganah And The Mossad Eliminated Jews, by Naeim Giladi... The painful truth about the Zionist rape of Palestine and deliberate planting of anti-Semitism in Iraqi Jewish communities during David Ben-Gurion's political career in order to persuade the Iraqi Jews to immigrate to Israel. (ISBN1-893302-40-7)

America, Awake! We Must Take Back Our Country, by Norman D. Livergood... This book is intended as a wake-up call for Americans, as Paul Revere awakened the Lexington patriots to the British attack on April 18, 1775, and as Thomas Paine's Common Sense roused apathetic American colonists to recognize and struggle against British oppression. Our current situation is similar to that which American patriots faced in the 1770s: a country ruled by 'foreign' and 'domestic' plutocratic powers and a divided citizenry uncertain of their vital interests. (ISBN 1-893302-27-X)

America's Nightmare: The Presidency of George Bush II, by John Stanton & Wayne Madsen...Media & Language, War & Weapons, Internal Affairs and a variety of other issues pointing out the US "crisis without precedent" that was wrought by the US Presidential election of 2000 followed by 9/11. "Stanton & Madsen will challenge many of the things you've been told by CNN and Fox news. This book is dangerous." (ISBN 1-893302-29-6)

America's Autopsy Report, by John Kaminski...The false fabric of history is unraveling beneath an avalanche of pathological lies to justify endless war and Orwellian new laws that revoke the rights of Americans. While TV and newspapers glorify the dangerous ideas of perverted billionaires, the Internet has pulsated with outrage and provided a new and real forum for freedom among concerned people all over the world who are opposed to the mass murder and criminal exploitation of the defenseless victims of multinational corporate totalitarianism. John Kaminski's passionate essays give voice to those hopes and fears of humane people that are ignored by the big business shysters who rule the major media. (ISBN 1-893302-42-3)

Seeds Of Fire: China And The Story Behind The Attack On America, by Gordon Thomas... The inside story about China that no one can afford to ignore. Using his unsurpassed contacts in Israel, Washington, London and Europe, Gordon Thomas, internationally acclaimed best-selling author and investigative reporter for over a quarter-century, reveals information about China's intentions to use the current crisis to launch itself as a super-power and become America's new major enemy..."This has been kept out of the news agenda because it does not suit certain business interests to have that truth emerge...Every patriotic American should buy and read this book... it is simply revelatory." (Ray Flynn, Former U.S. Ambassador to the Vatican) (ISBN 1-893302-54-7)

Shaking The Foundations: Coming Of Age In The Postmodern Era, by John H. Brand, D.Min., J.D.... Scientific discoveries in the Twentieth Century require the restructuring of our understanding the nature of Nature and of human beings. In simple language the author explains how significant implications of quantum mechanics, astronomy, biology and brain physiology form the foundation for new perspectives to comprehend the meaning of our lives. (ISBN 1-893302-25-3)

Rebuilding The Foundations: Forging A New And Just America, by John H. Brand, D.Min., J.D....Should we expect a learned scholar to warn us about our dangerous reptilian brains that are the real cause of today's evils? Although Brand is not without hope for rescuing America, he warns us to act fast–and now. Evil men intent on imposing their political, economic, and religious self-serving goals on America are not far from achieving their goal of mastery." (ISBN 1-893302-33-4)

The Last Days Of Israel, by Barry Chamish... With the Middle East crisis ongoing, *The Last Days of Israel* takes on even greater significance as an important book of our age. Barry Chamish, investigative reporter who has the true story about Yitzak Rabin's assassination, tells it like it is. (ISBN 1-893302-16-4)

Taboo: A Memoir – Confessions of Forbidden Love, by Tom Hathaway... A brave and honest exploration of the primal lust of our psyches, Taboo points the way to a new sexual frontier. Women who want to know what men really want must read this erotic rhapsody. A 21st century *Lady Chatterly's Lover* by a prolific new author whose name will soon become a household word. (ISBN 1-893302-87-3)

The Last Atlantis Book You'll Ever Have To Read! by Gene D. Matlock... More than 25,000 books, plus countless other articles have been written about a fabled confederation of city-states known as Atlantis. If it really did exist, where was it located? Does anyone have valid evidence of its existence – artifacts and other remnants? According to historian, archaeologist, educator and linguist Gene D. Matlock, both questions can easily be answered. (ISBN 1-893302-20-2)

Cancer Doctor: The Biography Josef Issels, M.D., Who Brought Hope To The World With His Revolutionary Cancer Treatment, by Gordon Thomas...Dr. Josef Issels treated more than 12,000 cancer patients who had been written off as "incurable" by other doctors. He claimed no miracle cures, but the success record of his revolutionary "whole person treatment" was extraordinary... the story of his struggle against the medical establishment which put Dr. Issels in prison, charged with fraud and manslaughter. (ISBN 1-893302-18-0)

ALL DANDELION BOOKS ARE AVAILABLE THROUGH WWW.DANDELIONBOOKS.NET... ALWAYS. NEW: TOLL-FREE ORDERS

1-800-861-7899 (U.S. & CANADA)

Printed in the United States
68412LVS00002B/284

9 781893 302969